THE
T-FACTOR
FAT GRAM
COUNTER

	DAY 1	2	3	4	5	6
Breakfast						
Snack						
Lunch						
Snack						
Dinner						
TOTAL						

	9	10	11	12	13	14	15	16	17	18	19	20	21

By Jamie Pope and Martin Katahn

The Low-Fat Fast Food Guide
The Low-Fat Supermarket Shopper's Guide
The T-Factor Fat Gram Counter

By Martin Katahn

How to Quit Smoking Without Gaining Weight
One Meal at a Time

By Martin Katahn and Terri Katahn

The Low-Fat Good Food Cookbook

THE T-FACTOR FAT GRAM COUNTER

COMPLETELY UP-TO-DATE

WITH 3-WEEK

RECORDING DIARY

JAMIE POPE, M.S., R.D.

MARTIN KATAHN, PH.D.

W. W. NORTON & COMPANY

NEW YORK LONDON

The text of this book is composed in Helvetica,
with the display set in Helvetica Bold.
Composition and manufacturing by MCUSA Inc.
Book design by Margaret Wagner.

ISBN 0-393-30655-0

W.W. Norton & Company, Inc.
500 Fifth Avenue, New York, N.Y. 10110
W. W. Norton & Company Ltd.
10 Coptic Street, London WC1A 1PU

    2 3 4 5 6 7 8 9 0

HOW TO USE THIS COUNTER

The food items in this counter are in alphabetical order within a number of different food categories.* The categories of foods are organized as follows, with the page number on which you will find them:

*Nutrient values in this counter were obtained from materials provided by the U.S. Department of Agriculture, as well as the food industry, journal articles, and computer data banks in which information is assumed to be public domain.

Foods are listed in commonly consumed portion sizes. Information is given for **total fat in grams, saturated fat in grams, milligrams (mg) of cholesterol, total calories, grams of fiber,** and **mg of sodium** (NA = not available). We have tried to include a wide sampling of foods and beverages. If you cannot find a product in this counter, consult the nutrition labeling that appears on food products or use the values of a similar food as an approximation. You can also write to the food company and request nutrition information. An extensive listing of virtually all low-fat brand-name foods can be found in *The Low-Fat Supermarket Shopper's Guide,* published by W. W. Norton and available at your local bookstore. Here we include many of the new "lite" and reduced-fat or -calorie products and an extensive list of combination foods. The latter includes representative items from different food manufacturers, or an average from several, without naming them. Combination foods may be listed as "hmde" (homemade) or "frzn" (frozen). Values for these dishes, soups, salads, and sandwiches represent combinations of ingredients from traditional recipes.

Values for total fat and saturated fat are presented to the nearest tenth of a gram in this counter. Government regulations permit food processors to round to the nearest whole gram on package labels. Thus, for example, a cereal product containing 0.3 gram of fat will be rounded down to 0 fat in the nutrition information presented on the carton, while another product containing 0.6 gram will be rounded up to 1.

We also include a wide sampling of items from fast-food chains and other popular restaurants with the most up-to-date information at the time of publication. Menu items are constantly changing, thus periodically request nutrition brochures and watch for new items at the fast-food establishments you frequently visit. *The Low-Fat Fast Food Guide,* also published by W. W. Norton, combines nutrition information for 30 national restaurant chains and is available at your local bookstore.

In the meat, fish, and poultry categories, values are for cooked portions, without added fat, unless otherwise specified. In some cases, where values vary according to cooking method, the cooking method is specified. Beef entries are grouped according to their percentage of total fat; the term "lean" refers to trimmed cuts with minimal marbling.

FAT-GRAM TOTALS FOR DIFFERENT PERCENTAGES
OF TOTAL CALORIES*

Total Calories	Grams of Total Fat Percentage of Total Calories:		
	20%	25%	30%
1,200	27	33	40
1,300	29	36	43
1,400	31	39	47
1,500	33	42	50
1,600	36	44	53
1,700	38	47	57
1,800	40	50	60
1,900	42	53	63
2,000	44	56	67
2,100	47	58	70
2,200	49	61	73
2,300	51	64	77
2,400	53	67	80
2,500	56	69	83
2,600	58	72	87
2,700	60	75	90

*Highly active persons of normal weight may need to consume more than 2,400 calories a day to maintain their weight. At higher levels of calorie intake, 25 and 30 percent of calories as fat go over our recommended upper levels of 50 and 60 grams per day for females and males, respectively. However, unless you are highly active (e.g., running 10 or more miles a day) or working in extremely cold or hot weather day after day (near zero or 100 degrees), there is no need to exceed our recommended upper limits of 50 and 60 grams of total fat per day. The additional figures have been added to the table for reference.

Item	Serving	Total Fat (g)	Saturated Fat (g)	Cholesterol (mg)	Calories	Fiber (g)	Sodium (mg)
BEVERAGES							
apple juice	6 fl. oz.	0	0	0	90	0	6
beer							
regular*	12 fl. oz.	0	0	0	148	0	19
light*	12 fl. oz.	0	0	0	100	0	10
nonalcoholic	12 fl. oz.	0	0	0	90	0	5
carbonated drink							
regular	12 fl. oz.	0	0	0	152	0	14
sugar free	12 fl. oz.	0	0	0	1	0	8
club soda/seltzer	12 fl. oz.	0	0	0	0	0	75
coffee, brewed or instant	8 fl. oz.	0	0	0	4	0	4
coffee, flavored mixes, instant	6 fl. oz.	2.4	1.9	0	55	0	192
cordials and liqueurs, 54 proof*	1 fl. oz.	0	0	0	97	0	3
daiquiri*	3.5 fl. oz.	0	0	0	122	0	0
eggnog, nonalcoholic							
w/whole milk	8 fl. oz.	19.0	11.2	149	342	0	138
w/2% fat milk	8 fl. oz.	8.1	3.8	194	188	0	155
fruit punch	8 fl. oz.	0	0	0	120	0	25
Gatorade sports drink	8 fl. oz.	0	0	0	60	0	96
gin*	1 fl. oz.	0	0	0	70	0	0
grape juice drink, canned	6 fl. oz.	0	0	0	89	0	12
Kool-Aid, from mix, any flavor	8 fl. oz.	0	0	0	95	0	8
lemonade, mix or frzn	8 fl. oz.	0	0	0	102	0	13
lemonade, sugar-free	8 fl. oz.	0	0	0	4	0	0

*Although alcohol contains no fat, scientific evidence suggests that it may facilitate fat storage and hamper your weight-loss efforts. Excessive alcohol intake is detrimental to your health. We concur with other health organizations in recommending discretion in the use of alcoholic beverages.

Item	Serving	Total Fat (g)	Saturated Fat (g)	Cholesterol (mg)	Calories	Fiber (g)	Sodium (mg)
orange juice, unsweetened	6 fl. oz.	0	0	0	83	0	2
pineapple-orange juice	6 fl. oz.	0	0	0	99	0	8
rum*	1 fl. oz.	0	0	0	70	0	0
Tang, orange or grape	8 fl. oz.	0	0	0	117	0	2
tea, brewed or instant	8 fl. oz.	0	0	0	0	0	3
tonic water	8 fl. oz.	0	0	0	90	0	10
vodka*	1 fl. oz.	0	0	0	70	0	0
whiskey*	1 fl. oz.	0	0	0	70	0	0
wine*							
dessert and apertif	4 fl. oz.	0	0	0	184	0	10
red or rosé	4 fl. oz.	0	0	0	85	0	0
white, dry or medium	4 fl. oz.	0	0	0	80	0	5
wine cooler	8 fl. oz.	0	0	0	83	0	9
BREADS AND FLOURS							
bagel, cinnamon raisin	1 medium	1.5	0.2	0	230	2	274
bagel, plain	1 medium	1.4	0.2	0	180	2	300
barley flour	1 cup	0.5	0.3	0	698	31	6
biscuit							
baking powder	1 medium	6.6	1.9	3	156	1	344
buttermilk	1 medium	4.8	1.2	2	103	1	366
from mix	1 medium	4.3	1.2	3	121	1	341
Bisquick mix	1 cup	17.0	4.1	0	511	2	1703
Boston brown bread							
canned	1/2-in. slice	0.6	0.2	0	85	2	100
w/raisins, canned	1/2-in. slice	0.6	0.2	0	88	2	130

*Although alcohol contains no fat, scientific evidence suggests that it may facilitate fat storage and hamper your weight-loss efforts. Excessive alcohol intake is detrimental to your health. We concur with other health organizations in recommending discretion in the use of alcoholic beverages.

Item	Serving	Total Fat (g)	Saturated Fat (g)	Cholesterol (mg)	Calories	Fiber (g)	Sodium (mg)
bread							
cracked wheat	1 slice	1.0	0.3	0	65	1	135
French/Vienna	1 slice	1.0	0.2	0	70	1	138
fruit w/nuts	1 slice	10.1	2.2	28	210	1	140
fruit w/o nuts	1 slice	5.9	1.5	22	150	1	110
honey wheatberry	1 slice	1.1	0.2	2	70	2	205
Italian	1 slice	0.5	0.1	0	78	1	151
mixed grain	1 slice	0.9	0.2	0	70	2	103
multigrain, "lite"	1 slice	0.5	0	2	45	3	117
pita, plain	1 large	0.8	0.1	0	240	2	430
pita, whole wheat	1 large	1.2	0.2	0	236	7	510
raisin	1 slice	1.0	0.2	1	70	1	94
Roman meal	1 slice	1.0	NA	5	68	1	57
rye, American	1 slice	0.9	0.2	0	66	2	174
rye, pumpernickel	1 slice	0.8	0.1	0	82	2	173
sourdough	1 slice	0.8	0.2	0	68	1	140
wheat, commercial	1 slice	1.1	0.3	0	75	1	151
wheat, "lite"	1 slice	0.5	0.1	0	45	3	118
white, commercial	1 slice	0.9	0.2	0	70	0	136
white, hmde	1 slice	1.7	0.3	10	72	0	102
white, "lite"	1 slice	0.5	0.1	0	42	2	91
whole wheat, commercial	1 slice	1.2	0.3	0	80	2	180
breadcrumbs	1 cup	4.6	1.1	0	392	3	736
breadsticks							
plain	1 small	0.2	0.1	0	23	0	70
sesame	1 small	3.7	1.2	0	56	0	85
bulgur, dry	1 cup	2.0	0.3	0	477	25	23
coffee cake	1 piece	7.0	2.1	19	233	1	160
cornbread							
from mix	1/8 mix	4.0	1.3	15	160	1	250
hmde	1 piece	7.3	2.2	17	198	2	232
cornflake crumbs	1 oz.	0	0	0	110	1	290

9

Item	Serving	Total Fat (g)	Saturated Fat (g)	Cholesterol (mg)	Calories	Fiber (g)	Sodium (mg)
cornmeal, dry	1 cup	1.6	0.3	0	502	10	201
cornstarch	1 T	0	0	0	35	0	0
crackers							
Captain's Wafers	2 crackers	1.0	0.4	0	30	0	88
cheese	5 pieces	4.9	1.6	4	81	0	180
Cheese Nips	13 crackers	3.0	1.1	3	70	0	130
cheese w/peanut butter	2 oz. pkg.	13.5	3.0	7	283	0	600
Chicken in a Biskit	7 crackers	4.0	1.2	3	70	0	115
Goldfish, any flavor	12 crackers	2.0	0.7	1	34	0	45
graham	2 squares	1.3	0.5	0	60	0	66
graham, crumbs	1/2 cup	4.5	2.0	1	180	2	180
Harvest Wheats	4 crackers	3.6	1.1	0	72	0	112
Hi Ho	4 crackers	4.4	1.3	1	82	0	31
matzohs	1 board	0.9	0.2	0	115	0	75
melba toast	1 piece	0.2	0	0	15	0	12
Norwegian flatbread	2 thin	0.3	0	0	40	0	32
oyster	33 crackers	3.3	0.7	0	120	0	250
Premium Fat Free	5 crackers	0	0	0	50	0	115
rice cakes	1 piece	0.3	0	0	35	0	10
rice wafer	3 wafers	0	0	0	31	0	195
Ritz	3 crackers	2.9	1.1	1	54	0	90
Ritz Bits	22 pieces	5.0	1.6	1	80	0	140
Ritz cheese	3 crackers	3.9	1.4	2	70	0	130
rye w/cheese	1.5 oz. pkg.	9.5	3.0	3	205	0	588
Ryekrisp, plain	2 crackers	0.2	0	0	50	0	100
Ryekrisp, sesame	2 crackers	1.5	0.4	0	60	0	141
saltines	2 crackers	0.6	0.1	0	26	0	80
sesame wafers	3 crackers	3.0	0.8	0	70	0	190
Snackwell's cheese	18 crackers	1.0	<1.0	0	60	NA	160
Snackwell's wheat	5 crackers	0	0	0	50	NA	160
Sociables	6 crackers	3.0	1.1	0	70	0	130
soda	5 crackers	1.6	0.4	0	42	0	156

Item	Serving	Total Fat (g)	Saturated Fat (g)	Cholesterol (mg)	Calories	Fiber (g)	Sodium (mg)
crackers *(cont.)*							
toasted w/peanut butter	1.5 oz. pkg.	10.5	2.9	2	212	0	405
Triscuit	2 crackers	1.3	0.2	0	42	0	60
Uneeda	2 crackers	1.0	0.3	0	42	0	67
Vegetable Thins	7 crackers	4.0	1.0	0	70	0	100
Wasa crispbread	1 piece	1.0	0.2	0	45	1	50
Waverly Wafers	2 crackers	1.6	0.6	0	36	0	80
Wheat Thins	4 crackers	1.4	0.5	0	36	0	60
Wheat Thins, nutty	4 crackers	2.8	0.9	0	45	0	142
wheat w/cheese	1.5 oz. pkg.	10.9	3.0	1	212	0	490
Wheatsworth	5 crackers	3.0	1.0	0	70	0	135
zwieback	2 crackers	0.7	0.2	0	40	0	20
crepe	1 medium	1.5	0.5	37	48	0	130
croissant	1 medium	11.5	6.9	30	167	1	126
croutons, commercial	1/4 cup	1.9	1.6	0	44	1	115
Danish pastry	1 medium	19.3	6.8	30	256	1	103
doughnut							
cake	1 2.2 oz.	16.2	4.1	24	250	1	229
yeast	1 2.2 oz.	13.3	5.2	21	235	1	222
dumpling, plain	1 medium	1.1	0.4	1	42	0	105
English muffin							
plain	1	1.1	0.2	0	135	1	291
w/raisins	1	1.2	0.2	0	150	1	203
whole wheat	1	2.5	0.5	0	139	2	147
flour							
buckwheat	1 cup	3.0	0.7	0	328	8	11
carob	1 cup	1.0	0.1	0	394	13	36
rice	1 cup	1.3	0.5	0	428	3	45
rye, medium	1 cup	1.5	0.2	0	308	13	1
soy	1 cup	18.0	2.5	0	380	2	11
wheat, cake	1 cup	0.8	0.1	0	349	4	2
white, all purpose	1 cup	1.2	0.2	0	418	4	2

Item	Serving	Total Fat (g)	Saturated Fat (g)	Cholesterol (mg)	Calories	Fiber (g)	Sodium (mg)
flour *(cont.)*							
white, bread	1 cup	1.2	0.2	0	409	4	2
white, self-rising	1 cup	1.2	0.2	0	436	4	1290
whole wheat	1 cup	2.4	0.3	0	399	11	4
French toast							
frzn variety	1 slice	6.0	1.0	54	139	0	257
hmde	1 slice	10.7	2.6	75	172	1	250
funnel cake	6 in. diam.	15.3	4.0	66	285	1	236
hushpuppy	1 medium	11.4	3.0	18	146	1	109
matzoh ball	1	7.6	2.2	76	121	0	202
muffins							
all types, commercial	1 large	10.3	4.3	24	187	1	263
banana nut	1 medium	5.0	2.2	20	135	2	175
blueberry, from mix	1 medium	4.3	1.9	9	126	0	185
bran, hmde	1 medium	5.1	2.1	16	112	2	160
corn	1 medium	4.2	1.2	18	130	1	192
white, plain	1 medium	4.0	2.2	12	118	0	132
pancakes							
blueberry, from mix	3 medium	15.0	4.3	85	320	4	438
buckwheat, from mix	3 medium	12.3	3.9	90	270	3	340
buttermilk, from mix	3 medium	10.0	3.2	105	270	2	463
hmde	3 medium	9.6	3.0	79	312	2	227
"lite," from mix	3 medium	2.0	NA	10	130	5	570
whole-wheat, from mix	3 medium	3.0	NA	NA	180	6	410
phyllo dough	2 oz.	3.4	0.5	0	170	1	274
pie crust, plain	1/8 pie	8.0	1.9	0	125	0	130
popover	1	5.0	2.6	51	170	0	176
rice bran	1 oz.	0.4	0.1	0	80	2	4
rolls							
brown & serve	1	2.2	<1.0	5	100	0	200
cloverleaf	1	3.2	0.6	21	89	0	155
crescent	1	5.6	2.8	6	102	1	256

Item	Serving	Total Fat (g)	Saturated Fat (g)	Cholesterol (mg)	Calories	Fiber (g)	Sodium (mg)
rolls *(cont.)*							
croissant	1 small	6.1	3.5	21	109	0	106
French	1	0.4	0.1	0	137	1	287
hamburger	1	3.0	0.8	1	180	1	304
hard	1	1.2	0.3	1	115	1	231
hot dog	1	2.1	0.5	1	116	1	241
kaiser/hoagie	1 medium	1.6	0.4	2	156	1	312
pan type	1 small	1.0	<0.5	0	80	0	140
parkerhouse	1	2.1	0.9	1	59	0	100
raisin	1 large	1.7	0.4	0	165	1	235
rye, dark	1	1.6	0.1	0	55	2	125
rye, light, hard	1	1.0	0.1	0	79	2	235
sandwich	1	3.1	0.4	2	162	1	312
sesame seed	1	2.1	0.6	1	59	1	210
sourdough	1	1.0	0	0	100	1	235
submarine	1 medium	3.0	0.8	3	290	2	580
wheat	1	1.7	0.4	0	52	1	130
white, commercial	1	2.0	1.0	1	110	0	175
white, hmde	1	3.1	0.5	2	119	1	202
whole wheat	1	1.1	0.2	1	85	3	184
yeast, sweet	1	7.9	2.1	20	198	1	106
scone	1	5.5	1.5	38	120	1	189
soft pretzel	1 medium	1.7	0.7	2	190	1	770
stuffing							
bread, from mix	1/2 cup	12.2	6.0	0	198	0	500
cornbread, from mix	1/2 cup	4.8	2.5	43	175	0	568
Stove Top	1/2 cup	9.0	5.0	21	176	0	560
sweet roll, iced	1 medium	7.9	2.1	20	198	1	100
toaster pastry, any flavor	1	5.0	0.8	0	195	0	229
tortilla							
corn (unfried)	1 medium	0.8	0.1	0	48	1	38
flour	1 medium	2.5	1.1	0	59	1	63

Item	Serving	Total Fat (g)	Saturated Fat (g)	Cholesterol (mg)	Calories	Fiber (g)	Sodium (mg)
turnover, fruit filled	1	15.0	3.7	0	280	1	260
waffle							
frozen, Eggo	1	5.0	1.0	15	120	1	250
frozen, other	1 medium	2.6	0.7	11	95	1	235
hmde	1 large	12.6	4.1	61	245	1	303
weiner wrap, plain/cheese	1 wrap	2.0	NA	NA	60	0	373

CANDY
Item	Serving	Total Fat (g)	Saturated Fat (g)	Cholesterol (mg)	Calories	Fiber (g)	Sodium (mg)
butterscotch							
candy	6 pieces	2.5	0.5	0	116	0	19
chips	1 oz.	6.7	NA	0	234	0	15
candied fruit							
apricot	1 oz.	0.1	0	0	94	1	5
cherry	1 oz.	0.1	0	0	96	1	5
citrus peel	1 oz.	0.1	0	0	90	1	5
figs	1 oz.	0.1	0	0	84	2	5
candy bar							
Almond Joy	1 oz.	7.8	5.3	1	136	2	58
Baby Ruth	1 oz.	6.6	2.4	1	141	1	60
Bit-o-Honey	1 oz.	2.2	NA	NA	121	0	80
Butterfinger	1 oz.	5.5	2.6	0	131	1	46
Chunky	1 oz.	8.3	6.6	3	140	1	15
Golden Almond, Hershey	1 oz.	11.0	2.1	5	161	2	17
Heath	1 oz.	8.9	4.1	2	142	1	109
Kit Kat	1.13 oz.	9.2	5.3	8	162	0	32
Krackle, Hershey	1 oz.	8.4	4.7	5	145	1	35
Mars	1.7 oz.	11.0	4.6	4	230	1	80
milk choc., Hershey	1 oz.	9.2	5.0	6	147	1	27
milk choc., Nestle	1 oz.	9.0	5.0	6	146	1	18
milk choc. w/almonds	1 oz.	10.1	4.8	5	151	2	17
Milky Way	1 oz.	3.9	2.2	2	118	0	49
Mounds	1 oz.	7.3	5.3	0	131	2	52

Item	Serving	Total Fat (g)	Saturated Fat (g)	Cholesterol (mg)	Calories	Fiber (g)	Sodium (mg)
candy bar *(cont.)*							
Mr. Goodbar	1 oz.	10.8	4.7	4	154	2	19
Nestle's Crunch	1.06 oz.	8.0	4.5	4	160	1	35
Snickers	1 oz.	6.5	3.0	3	135	1	75
Special Dark, Hershey	1.02 oz.	8.6	NA	NA	157	1	5
Three Musketeers	1 oz.	4.0	1.8	2	140	0	67
Twix	1 oz.	7.0	NA	3	140	0	60
candy-coated almonds	1 oz.	5.3	0.4	0	129	1	6
caramels							
plain or choc. w/nuts	1 oz.	6.9	2.5	10	120	0	10
plain or choc. w/o nuts	1 oz.	5.8	2.4	9	114	0	10
carob-coated raisins	1/2 cup	13.5	1.9	0	387	5	83
choc. chips							
milk choc.	1/4 cup	11.0	6.2	0	218	1	60
semi-sweet	1/4 cup	12.2	6.9	0	220	1	10
choc.-covered cherries	1 oz.	4.9	2.9	1	123	1	52
choc.-covered cream center	1 oz.	4.9	2.6	1	123	1	52
choc.-covered mint patty	1 small	1.0	0.6	0	40	0	3
choc.-covered peanuts	1 oz.	11.7	4.6	0	159	2	17
choc.-covered raisins	1 oz.	4.9	2.9	3	120	1	18
choc.kisses	6 pieces	9.0	5.0	6	154	1	25
choc. stars	7 pieces	8.1	4.7	5	160	1	35
Cracker Jack	1 cup	3.3	0.4	0	170	2	125
creme eggs, Cadbury	1 oz.	6.0	NA	NA	136	0	NA
English toffee	1 oz.	2.8	1.7	5	113	0	8
fondant	1 piece	0.2	0.2	0	116	0	52
fudge							
choc.	1 oz.	3.4	1.5	1	112	0	45
choc. w/nuts	1 oz.	4.9	1.2	1	119	0	48
Good & Plenty	1 oz.	0.1	0	0	106	0	10
gumdrops	28 pieces	0.2	0	0	97	0	15
Gummy Bears	1 oz.	0.1	0	0	110	0	13

Item	Serving	Total Fat (g)	Saturated Fat (g)	Cholesterol (mg)	Calories	Fiber (g)	Sodium (mg)
hard candy	6 pieces	0.3	0	0	108	0	9
jelly beans	1 oz.	0	0	0	104	0	3
licorice	1 oz.	0.1	0	0	35	0	10
Life Savers	5 pieces	0.1	0	0	39	0	1
M&M's							
choc. only	1 oz.	5.6	2.4	3	132	1	20
peanut	1 oz.	7.8	2.4	4	145	1	18
malted-milk balls	1 oz.	7.1	4.2	3	137	1	28
marshmallow	1 large	0	0	0	25	0	0
marshmallow cremes	1 oz.	0.1	0	0	88	0	13
mints	14 pieces	0.6	0	0	104	0	10
peanut brittle	1 oz.	7.7	1.2	0	149	1	44
Peanut Butter Cups,							
Reese's	1 oz.	9.2	3.6	3	156	1	82
Peppermint Pattie	1 oz.	4.8	2.6	1	124	1	52
praline	1 oz.	6.9	0.5	0	130	0	18
Reese's Pieces	1.7 oz. pkg.	13.0	NA	2	240	0	108
sour balls	1 oz.	0	0	0	110	0	15
Starburst fruit chews	1 oz.	2.4	NA	0	112	0	16
Sugar Daddy caramel	1.4 oz.	1.0	NA	NA	150	0	85
taffy	1 oz.	1.5	0.4	0	99	0	131
Tootsie Roll pop	1 oz.	0.6	0.2	0	110	0	1
Tootsie Roll	1 oz.	2.3	0.6	0	112	1	56
yogurt-covered peanuts	1/2 cup	26.0	5.1	3	387	4	30
yogurt-covered raisins	1/2 cup	14.0	11.4	2	313	2	36
CEREALS							
All Bran	3/4 cup	1.1	0.2	0	159	19	719
Alpha-Bits	1 cup	0.6	0.2	0	111	1	170
Apple Jacks	1 cup	0.1	0	0	110	1	200
Bran, 100%	1/2 cup	1.9	0.3	0	84	9	189
bran, unprocessed, dry	1/4 cup	0.6	0.1	0	29	6	1

Item	Serving	Total Fat (g)	Saturated Fat (g)	Cholesterol (mg)	Calories	Fiber (g)	Sodium (mg)
Bran Buds	1/3 cup	0.7	0.1	0	72	10	172
Bran Chex	1 cup	1.2	0.2	0	136	9	448
Bran Flakes, 40%	1 cup	0.7	0.1	0	127	6	303
Cap'n Crunch	3/4 cup	3.4	1.7	0	121	0	185
Cheerios	1 cup	1.6	0.3	0	90	2	233
Cocoa Krispies	1 cup	0.5	0.2	0	140	0	275
Corn Chex	1 cup	0.1	0	0	111	1	271
cornflakes	1 cup	0.1	0	0	108	1	279
corn grits w/o added fat	1/2 cup	0.5	0	0	71	1	0
Cracklin' Oat Bran	1/3 cup	2.7	1.3	0	72	3	116
Cream of Wheat w/o added fat	1/2 cup	0.3	0	0	67	0	3
Crispix	1 cup	0	0	0	110	1	220
Fiber One	1 cup	2.2	0.4	0	128	21	463
Fiberwise	2/3 cup	1.0	0	0	90	5	140
Frosted Bran, Kellogg's	2/3 cup	0	0	0	100	3	190
Frosted Mini-Wheats	4 biscuits	0.3	0	0	102	1	8
Fruit & Fibre w/apples & cinn.	1/2 cup	0.3	0	0	90	3	160
w/dates, raisins, walnuts	1/2 cup	0.7	0.1	0	89	4	162
Fruit Loops	1 cup	0	0	0	111	1	200
fruit squares, Kellogg's	1/2 cup	0	0	0	90	2	5
Fruitful Bran	2/3 cup	0	0	0	120	5	240
Golden Grahams	3/4 cup	1.1	0.1	0	109	1	178
granola commercial brands	1/3 cup	6.9	3.3	0	186	3	58
hmde	1/3 cup	10.0	4.8	0	184	2	80
low-fat, Kellogg's	1/3 cup	2.0	0	0	120	2	60
Grapenut Flakes	1 cup	0.4	0.2	0	116	2	158
Grapenuts	1/4 cup	0.2	0	0	104	2	188
Honeynut Cheerios	3/4 cup	0.7	0.1	0	107	1	250

Item	Serving	Total Fat (g)	Saturated Fat (g)	Cholesterol (mg)	Calories	Fiber (g)	Sodium (mg)
Kix	1 1/2 cup	0.7	0.2	0	110	0	290
Life, plain or cinn.	1 cup	2.6	0.5	0	162	4	241
Most	2/3 cup	0.3	0	0	95	2	150
Mueslix, Kellogg's	1/2 cup	1.0	0.8	0	140	4	94
Nutri-Grain, Kellogg's							
almond raisin	2/3 cup	2.0	0	0	140	3	220
raisin bran	1 cup	1.0	0	0	130	5	200
wheat	2/3 cup	0.3	0	0	90	3	170
oat bran, cooked cereal							
w/o added fat	1/2 cup	1.2	0.4	0	55	2	256
oat bran, dry	1/4 cup	1.6	0.3	0	82	3	1
oats							
instant	1 packet	1.7	0.2	0	108	1	105
w/o added fat	1/2 cup	1.2	0.2	0	72	1	1
Product 19	1 cup	0.2	0	0	108	1	325
puffed rice	1 cup	0	0	0	56	0	0
puffed wheat	1 cup	0.1	0	0	44	1	1
Raisin Bran	1 cup	0.8	0.1	0	156	5	296
Rice Chex	1 cup	0.1	0	0	111	1	271
Rice Krispies	1 cup	0.2	0	0	110	0	291
shredded wheat	1 cup	0.5	0.1	0	85	2	3
Shredded Wheat Squares,							
fruit filled	1/2 cup	0	0	0	90	3	5
Special K	1 cup	0.1	0	0	111	0	265
Sugar Frosted Flakes	1 cup	0	0	0	147	1	267
Sugar Smacks	3/4 cup	0.5	0	0	106	1	70
Team	1 cup	0.5	0.1	0	111	1	175
Total	1 cup	0.7	0.1	0	100	2	280
Total raisin bran	1 cup	1.0	0.1	0	140	5	190
Wheat Chex	1 cup	1.2	0.2	0	169	6	308
wheat germ, toasted	1/4 cup	3.0	0.5	0	108	4	1
Wheaties	1 cup	0.5	0.1	0	99	2	270

Item	Serving	Total Fat (g)	Saturated Fat (g)	Cholesterol (mg)	Calories	Fiber (g)	Sodium (mg)
whole-wheat, natural, w/o added fat	1/2 cup	0.7	0.1	0	71	2	10

CHEESES

Item	Serving	Total Fat (g)	Saturated Fat (g)	Cholesterol (mg)	Calories	Fiber (g)	Sodium (mg)
Alpine Lace, Free 'n' Lean							
American	1 oz.	0	0	5	35	0	290
cheddar	1 oz.	0	0	5	35	0	290
mozzarella	1 oz.	0	0	5	35	0	290
American							
processed	1 oz.	8.9	5.6	27	106	0	406
reduced calorie	1 oz.	2.2	2.3	12	50	0	400
blue	1 oz.	8.2	5.3	21	100	3	396
Borden's Fat Free	1 oz.	<9.5	NA	<5	40	0	380
Borden's Lite Line	1 oz.	2.0	NA	NA	50	0	420
brick	1 oz.	8.4	5.3	27	105	0	159
Brie	1 oz.	7.9	4.9	28	95	0	178
caraway	1 oz.	8.3	5.4	30	107	0	196
cheddar							
grated	1/4 cup	9.4	6.0	30	114	0	176
sliced	1 oz.	9.4	6.0	30	114	0	176
cheese fondue	1/4 cup	11.7	7.2	37	170	0	109
cheese food, cold pack	2 T	7.8	4.4	18	94	0	274
cheese sauce	1/4 cup	9.8	4.3	20	132	0	576
cheese spread (Kraft)	1 oz.	6.0	3.8	16	82	0	381
Cheez Whiz	1 oz.	6.0	3.1	16	80	0	370
Colby	1 oz.	9.1	5.7	27	112	0	171
cottage cheese							
1% fat	1/2 cup	1.2	0.8	5	82	0	459
2% fat	1/2 cup	2.2	1.4	10	101	0	459
creamed	1/2 cup	5.1	3.2	17	117	0	457
cream cheese							
Kraft Free	1 oz. (2T)	0	0	5	25	0	390

Item	Serving	Total Fat (g)	Saturated Fat (g)	Cholesterol (mg)	Calories	Fiber (g)	Sodium (mg)
cream cheese *(cont.)*							
"lite" (Neufchâtel)	1 oz. (2T)	6.6	4.2	20	74	0	113
regular	1 oz. (2T)	9.9	6.2	31	99	0	84
Weight Watchers	1 oz. (2T)	2.0	NA	NA	35	0	40
Edam	1 oz.	7.9	5.0	25	101	0	274
feta	1 oz.	6.0	4.2	25	75	0	316
Gouda	1 oz.	7.8	5.0	32	101	0	232
Healthy Choice	1 oz.	0	0	5	30	0	390
hot pepper cheese	1 oz.	6.9	4.3	18	92	0	357
Jarlsberg	1 oz.	6.9	4.2	16	100	0	130
Kraft American Singles	1 oz.	7.0	4.0	25	90	0	390
Kraft Free Singles	1 oz.	0	0	5	45	0	430
Kraft Light Singles	1 oz.	4.0	2.0	15	70	0	410
Light n' Lively singles	1 oz.	4.0	2.0	15	70	0	400
Limburger	1 oz.	7.7	4.8	26	93	0	227
Monterey Jack	1 oz.	8.6	5.0	30	106	0	152
mozzarella							
part skim	1 oz.	4.5	2.4	16	72	0	132
part skim, low moisture	1 oz.	4.9	3.1	15	79	0	150
whole milk	1 oz.	6.1	3.7	22	80	0	106
whole milk, low moisture	1 oz.	7.0	4.4	25	90	0	118
Muenster	1 oz.	8.5	5.4	27	104	0	178
Parmesan							
grated	1 T	1.5	1.0	4	23	0	93
hard	1 oz.	7.3	4.7	19	111	0	454
Weight Watchers Fat Free	1 T	0	0	0	14	0	60
pimento cheese spread	1 oz.	9.4	5.6	27	106	0	405
port wine, cold pack	1 oz.	9.0	4.7	35	100	0	151
provolone	1 oz	7.6	4.8	20	100	0	248
ricotta							
"lite" reduced fat	1/2 cup	4.0	NA	15	109	0	132
part skim	1/2 cup	9.8	6.1	38	171	0	155

Item	Serving	Total Fat (g)	Saturated Fat (g)	Cholesterol (mg)	Calories	Fiber (g)	Sodium (mg)
ricotta *(cont.)*							
whole milk	1/2 cup	16.1	10.3	63	216	0	104
Romano	1 oz.	7.6	4.9	29	110	0	340
Roquefort	1 oz.	8.7	5.5	26	105	0	513
Sargento Preferred Light							
mozzarella	1 oz.	3.0	2.0	10	60	0	150
Swiss	1 oz.	4.0	3.0	15	80	0	75
smoked cheese product	1 oz.	6.7	NA	20	91	0	220
Swiss							
processed	1 oz.	7.1	2.9	15	95	0	388
sliced	1 oz.	7.8	5.0	26	107	0	74
Velveeta	1 oz.	7.0	4.0	20	100	0	410
Velveeta Light	1 oz.	4.0	2.0	15	70	0	470
Weight Watchers, slices	1 oz.	2.0	1.0	15	50	0	400
COMBINATION FOODS							
baked beans w/ pork	1/2 cup	1.8	0.8	8	134	4	524
beans & franks, canned	1 cup	16.0	6.0	15	366	7	1105
beans							
refried, canned	1/2 cup	1.4	0.5	0	135	7	530
refried w/fat	1/2 cup	13.2	5.2	12	271	7	1071
refried w/sausage, canned	1/2 cup	13.0	6.0	25	194	8	825
beef & vegetable stew	1 cup	10.5	4.9	64	218	2	292
beef burgundy	1 cup	21.2	8.0	72	336	1	467
beef goulash w/noodles	1 cup	13.9	3.6	87	335	2	453
beef noodle casserole	1 cup	19.2	6.5	81	329	2	1205
beef pot pie							
frzn	8 oz.	23.0	5.9	41	430	2	1093
hmde	8 oz.	30.0	8.0	42	515	3	596
beef stew, canned	1 cup	8.0	2.4	34	184	2	977
beef teriyaki, Stouffer's	10 oz.	8.0	NA	NA	290	2	1450
beef vegetable stew, hmde	1 cup	13.8	5.3	46	244	2	649

Item	Serving	Total Fat (g)	Saturated Fat (g)	Cholesterol (mg)	Calories	Fiber (g)	Sodium (mg)
beef							
chipped, creamed	1/2 cup	11.0	3.7	21	175	0	681
short ribs w/gravy, frzn	5 3/4 oz.	25.0	10.0	59	350	0	702
burrito							
bean w/cheese	1 large	9.7	5.4	26	230	4	642
bean w/o cheese	1 large	2.8	0.9	3	142	4	510
beef	1 large	24.9	10.1	86	424	2	712
with guacamole, frzn	6 oz.	16.0	NA	NA	354	2	823
cabbage roll w/beef & rice	1 medium	8.2	2.9	26	172	2	386
cannelloni, meat & cheese	1 piece	29.7	13.5	185	420	1	597
casserole, meat, veg., rice,							
sauce	1 cup	12.2	4.7	62	276	3	238
cheese soufflé	1 cup	11.0	3.2	132	174	0	118
chicken, glazed, Lean							
Cuisine	8 1/2 oz.	8.0	2.0	55	260	1	570
chicken à la king, hmde	1 cup	34.3	12.7	186	468	1	760
chicken à la king w/ rice,							
frzn	1 cup	21.9	7.9	122	420	10	1016
chicken & dumplings	1 cup	10.5	2.7	103	298	1	611
chicken & rice casserole	1 cup	18.0	5.1	103	365	1	600
chicken & veg. stir-fry	1 cup	6.9	1.2	26	142	3	482
chicken cacciatore,							
Stouffer's	11 1/4 oz.	11.0	NA	NA	310	1	770
chicken divan, Stouffer's	8 1/2 oz.	20.0	NA	NA	320	0	780
chicken fricassee, hmde	1 cup	20.9	7.2	85	328	1	370
chicken-fried steak	3 1/2 oz.	23.4	6.8	115	355	0	365
chicken noodle casserole	1 cup	10.7	3.2	59	269	2	866
chicken parmigiana, hmde	7 oz.	14.8	4.5	11	308	2	620
chicken pot pie							
frzn	8 oz.	23.0	7.6	40	430	1	906
hmde	8 oz.	31.4	10.3	56	546	2	594
chicken salad, regular	1/2 cup	21.2	9.1	56	271	0	316

Item	Serving	Total Fat (g)	Saturated Fat (g)	Cholesterol (mg)	Calories	Fiber (g)	Sodium (mg)
chicken tetrazzini	1 cup	19.6	6.9	50	348	1	813
chicken w/cashews, Chinese	1 cup	10.9	2.3	22	203	3	1228
chili							
w/beans	1 cup	14.8	5.9	52	302	6	915
w/o beans	1 cup	19.3	7.8	70	302	3	1030
chitterlings, cooked	3 1/2 oz.	29.4	10.1	143	303	0	39
chop suey w/o rice							
beef	1 cup	17.0	8.5	55	300	3	1053
fish or poultry	1 cup	6.7	1.7	10	124	4	1564
chow mein							
beef, canned, La Choy	1 cup	2.3	NA	NA	72	2	900
chicken, canned, La Choy	1 cup	2.3	NA	NA	68	2	800
chicken, hmde	1 cup	8.8	2.4	75	224	2	718
pepper, La Choy	1 cup	1.4	NA	NA	89	2	720
corned-beef hash	1 cup	24.4	7.5	80	374	2	1158
crab cake	1 small	3.8	1.4	39	61	0	132
creamed chipped beef	1 cup	22.0	7.8	55	332	0	1608
curry w/o meat	1 cup	6.6	2.8	15	138	2	294
deviled crab	1/2 cup	15.4	4.1	50	231	1	468
deviled egg	1 large	5.3	1.2	109	63	0	140
egg foo yung w/sauce	1 piece	11.5	3.0	107	129	1	492
egg salad	1/2 cup	17.4	3.7	327	212	0	354
eggplant Parmesan, traditional	1 cup	24.0	8.7	31	356	3	1196
egg roll							
restaurant	1 (3 1/2 oz.)	10.5	2.6	52	153	1	469
frzn, La Choy	4	4.5	NA	NA	112	1	168
enchilada							
bean, beef, & cheese	1 piece	14.1	7.3	38	243	3	756
beef, frzn	7 1/2 oz.	16.0	NA	NA	250	1	1200

Item	Serving	Total Fat (g)	Saturated Fat (g)	Cholesterol (mg)	Calories	Fiber (g)	Sodium (mg)
enchilada *(cont.)*							
cheese, frzn	8 oz.	21.0	NA	NA	366	1	1175
chicken, frzn	7 1/2 oz.	11.0	NA	NA	247	1	1105
fajitas							
chicken	1	13.5	3.0	41	381	4	363
beef	1	18.2	6.1	34	302	3	761
falafel	1 small	5.0	0.8	9	74	1	36
fettuccine Alfredo	1 cup	29.7	NA	NA	461	1	912
fillet of fish divan, frzn	12 3/8 oz.	3.0	NA	85	240	0	700
fish creole	1 cup	5.4	NA	NA	172	2	NA
fritter, corn	1 medium	8.5	2.0	0	132	1	167
frzn dinner							
chopped beefsteak	11 oz.	26.5	NA	NA	443	2	NA
chopped steak	18 oz.	41.0	NA	NA	730	3	NA
fried chicken	11 oz.	31.0	NA	NA	590	2	1831
meat loaf	19 oz.	57.7	NA	NA	916	3	3050
meat loaf	11 oz.	29.0	NA	NA	530	2	1525
Salisbury steak	11 oz.	29.0	NA	NA	500	2	1340
turkey	11 oz.	11.0	NA	NA	360	2	1416
green pepper stuffed							
w/rice & beef	1 average	13.5	5.8	52	262	2	986
ham salad w/mayo	1/2 cup	20.2	4.4	54	277	0	1300
ham spread, Spreadables	1/2 cup	19.7	10.4	45	271	0	1156
Hamburger Helper, all							
varieties	1 cup	18.9	7.2	76	375	1	1037
hamburger rice casserole	1 cup	21.0	7.7	57	376	3	755
lasagna							
cheese, frzn	10 1/2 oz.	14.0	NA	NA	385	2	800
hmde w/beef & cheese	1 piece	19.8	10.0	81	400	2	1316
zucchini lasagna, Lean							
Cuisine	11 oz.	5.0	2.0	20	260	2	550
lo mein, Chinese	1 cup	7.2	1.4	11	185	1	368

Item	Serving	Total Fat (g)	Saturated Fat (g)	Cholesterol (mg)	Calories	Fiber (g)	Sodium (mg)
lobster							
Cantonese	1 cup	19.6	5.6	240	334	0	1586
Newburg	1/2 cup	24.8	14.7	183	305	0	670
salad	1/2 cup	7.0	1.5	36	119	0	432
macaroni & cheese							
from package	1 cup	17.3	6.0	22	386	0	1087
frzn	6 oz.	12.0	NA	17	260	0	800
manicotti, cheese & tomato	1 piece	11.8	6.0	61	238	2	610
meatball (reg. ground beef)	1 medium	5.1	2.0	30	72	0	94
meat loaf, w/reg. ground beef	3 1/2 oz.	20.4	8.5	102	332	0	696
moo goo gai pan	1 cup	17.2	3.1	66	304	1	595
moussaka	1 cup	8.9	2.8	98	210	3	400
onion rings	10 average	17.0	6.0	0	234	1	263
oysters Rockefeller, traditional	6-8 oysters	14.0	4.6	75	230	1	900
pepper steak	1 cup	21.3	4.4	73	329	1	649
pizza							
cheese	1 slice	10.1	5.2	40	183	1	680
cheese, French bread, frzn	5 1/8 oz.	13.0	6.7	37	330	1	840
combination w/meat	1 slice	17.5	9.0	56	272	1	1000
deep dish, cheese	1 slice	13.5	6.9	45	426	4	1170
pepperoni, frzn	1/4 pizza	18.0	9.3	47	364	2	825
pizza rolls, Jeno's	3 pieces	6.9	2.0	10	129	1	229
pork, sweet & sour, w/rice	1 cup	7.5	2.0	31	270	1	860
quiche							
Lorraine (bacon)	1/8 pie	43.5	20.1	218	540	1	567
plain or vegetable	1 slice	17.6	NA	135	312	1	539
ratatouille	1/2 cup	7.5	NA	0	87	2	880
ravioli, canned	1 cup	7.3	3.6	20	240	3	1002

Item	Serving	Total Fat (g)	Saturated Fat (g)	Cholesterol (mg)	Calories	Fiber (g)	Sodium (mg)
ravioli w/meat & tomato sauce	1 piece	3.0	0.9	19	49	0	96
Salisbury steak w/ gravy	8 oz.	27.3	12.3	126	364	1	1261
salmon patty, traditional	3 1/2 oz.	12.4	4.1	94	239	1	783
sandwiches							
BBQ beef on bun	1	16.8	5.8	54	392	5	1056
BBQ pork on bun	1	12.2	3.7	56	359	5	895
BLT w/mayo	1	15.6	4.1	23	282	1	935
bologna & cheese	1	22.5	9.7	42	363	1	1010
chicken w/mayo & lettuce	1	14.4	1.8	119	303	1	256
club w/mayo	1	20.8	5.4	52	590	3	1396
corned beef on rye	1	10.8	3.2	34	296	1	774
cream cheese & jelly	1	16.0	10.8	38	368	1	421
egg salad	1	12.5	2.5	228	279	1	482
french dip, au jus	1	12.2	4.8	58	360	2	610
grilled cheese	1	24.0	12.4	56	426	1	1177
ham, cheese & mayo	1	9.8	2.3	29	281	1	412
ham salad	1	16.9	4.2	40	321	1	372
peanut butter & jelly	1	15.1	2.3	10	374	3	406
Reuben	1	33.3	11.8	77	531	6	1535
roast beef & gravy	1	24.5	NA	55	429	1	785
roast beef & mayo	1	22.6	NA	60	328	1	800
sloppy joe on bun	1	16.8	5.8	54	392	5	1056
sub w/salami & cheese	1	41.3	17.7	109	766	3	1842
tuna salad	1	14.2	1.3	10	278	1	443
turkey & mayo	1	18.4	1.9	17	402	1	517
turkey breast & mustard	1	5.2	1.2	15	285	1	473
turkey ham on rye	1	9.0	1.9	34	239	3	986
shepherd's pie	1 cup	24.0	7.6	41	407	3	1158
shrimp creole w/o rice	1 cup	6.1	1.2	123	146	2	962
shrimp salad	1/2 cup	9.5	1.6	69	136	1	1087

Item	Serving	Total Fat (g)	Saturated Fat (g)	Cholesterol (mg)	Calories	Fiber (g)	Sodium (mg)
spaghetti							
w/meat sauce	1 cup	16.7	5.0	56	317	2	1320
w/red clam sauce	1 cup	7.3	1.0	17	250	2	306
w/white clam sauce	1 cup	19.5	2.6	49	416	1	436
w/tomato sauce	1 cup	1.5	0.4	5	179	2	910
SpaghettiOs, Franco American	1 cup	2.0	NA	NA	160	2	910
spanakopita	1 piece	24.1	7.0	79	259	2	354
spinach soufflé	1 cup	14.8	7.1	184	212	2	763
stroganoff							
beef, Stouffer's	9 3/4 oz.	20.0	NA	72	390	1	1090
beef w/o noodles	1 cup	44.4	19.4	8	568	1	634
sushi w/fish & vegetables	5 oz.	1.0	0.2	10	210	1	250
taco, beef	1 medium	17.0	8.5	54	272	2	355
tamale w/sauce	1 piece	6.0	1.6	3	114	1	356
tortellini, meat or cheese	1 cup	15.4	5.4	238	363	1	764
tostada w/refried beans	1 medium	16.3	6.7	20	294	6	249
Tuna Helper	1 cup	9.7	2.1	30	295	1	866
tuna noodle casserole	1 cup	13.3	3.1	38	315	2	109
tuna salad							
oil pack, w/mayo	1/2 cup	16.3	2.7	20	226	0	351
water pack, w/mayo	1/2 cup	10.5	1.6	14	170	0	112
veal parmigiana							
hmde	1 cup	25.5	9.2	102	485	2	1028
frzn	5 oz.	16.2	NA	67	287	0	858
veal scallopini	1 cup	20.4	7.3	132	429	2	160
Welsh rarebit	1 cup	31.6	17.3	NA	415	0	770
wonton w/pork, fried	1 piece	4.3	1.1	21	82	0	147
Yorkshire pudding	1 piece	2.4	1.0	30	56	0	83
DESSERTS AND TOPPINGS							
apple betty, fruit crisps	1/2 cup	13.3	2.7	0	347	3	114

Item	Serving	Total Fat (g)	Saturated Fat (g)	Cholesterol (mg)	Calories	Fiber (g)	Sodium (mg)
baklava	1 piece	29.2	7.2	7	426	2	288
brownie							
butterscotch	1	1.8	0.7	8	52	0	22
choc., "light," from mix	1/24 pkg.	2.0	<1.0	10	100	0	80
choc., Little Debbie	2 small	7.3	NA	NA	219	0	135
choc., plain	1 small	3.4	1.5	14	64	0	42
choc., w/nuts & icing	1	5.0	1.3	NA	64	0	40
Hostess	1 small	6.0	NA	NA	151	0	50
Pepperidge Farm	1	8.7	NA	NA	168	0	70
cake							
angel food	1/12 cake	0.2	0	0	161	0	161
banana w/frosting	1/12 cake	16.0	2.7	60	410	1	290
black forest	1/12 cake	14.3	2.1	57	279	1	150
butter w/frosting	1/12 cake	13.0	1.9	61	380	1	400
carrot w/frosting	1/12 cake	19.0	3.8	66	420	3	197
choc. w/frosting	1/12 cake	17.0	4.2	87	388	2	648
coconut w/frosting	1/12 cake	18.1	5.9	53	395	2	177
devil's food, "light," from mix	1/12 cake	3.5	1.5	45	190	0	350
German choc. w/frosting	1/12 cake	18.5	4.4	82	407	2	600
gingerbread	2 1/2" slice	2.9	1.8	2	267	0	225
lemon chiffon	1/12 cake	4.0	0.8	5	190	0	15
lemon w/frosting	1/12 cake	16.0	2.8	61	410	1	160
marble w/frosting	1/12 cake	16.0	2.9	69	408	1	172
pineapple upside-down	2 1/2" slice	9.2	1.9	48	236	2	165
pound	1/12 cake	9.0	4.4	53	200	1	110
pound, Entenmann fat-free	1 oz. slice	0	0	0	70	0	100
shortbread w/fruit	1 piece	8.9	2.1	60	344	1	165
spice w/frosting	1/12 cake	10.9	2.3	52	325	1	155
sponge	1 piece	3.7	0	137	194	0	210

Item	Serving	Total Fat (g)	Saturated Fat (g)	Cholesterol (mg)	Calories	Fiber (g)	Sodium (mg)
cake *(cont.)*							
streusel swirl	1/12 cake	11.0	2.0	40	260	1	163
white w/frosting	1/12 cake	14.6	3.6	5	369	1	420
white, "light," from mix	1/12 cake	3.0	1.0	20	180	0	320
yellow w/frosting	1/12 cake	16.4	5.9	55	391	1	108
yellow, "light," from mix	1/12 cake	3.5	1.5	45	190	0	300
cheesecake, traditional	1/8 pie	22.0	10.4	36	372	0	455
cobbler							
w/biscuit topping	1/2 cup	6.0	1.7	2	209	3	208
w/pie-crust topping	1/2 cup	9.3	3.6	5	236	3	151
cookie							
animal	15 cookies	4.7	1.2	0	152	0	134
anise-seed	1	4.0	1.6	8	63	0	30
anisette toast	1 slice	3.4	0.6	21	95	0	81
arrowroot	1	0.9	<1.0	<2	24	0	28
Bordeaux, Pepperidge Farm	1	1.8	1.0	0	39	0	32
Capri, Pepperidge Farm	1	4.6	1.0	0	82	0	45
Chantilly, Pepperidge Farm	1	2.0	1.0	<5	80	0	35
choc.	1	3.3	1.0	6	56	0	43
choc. chip, hmde	1	3.7	2.0	8	68	0	26
choc. chip, Pepperidge Farm	1 large	6.4	2.0	5	130	0	60
choc. sandwich (Oreo type)	1	2.1	0	0	49	0	0
Entenmann's fat free	2	0	0	0	75	0	115
fat-free Newtons	1	0	0	0	70	0	95
fig bar	1	0.9	0.3	6	56	1	40
Fig Newtons	1	1.0	<1.0	0	60	0	60
gingersnap	1	1.6	0.3	0	34	0	40

Item	Serving	Total Fat (g)	Saturated Fat (g)	Cholesterol (mg)	Calories	Fiber (g)	Sodium (mg)
graham cracker, choc. covered	1	3.1	0.9	0	62	0	53
Health Valley fat-free	3	0	0	0	75	2	40
Lido, Pepperidge Farm	1	5.3	1.0	4	90	0	40
macaroon, coconut	1	1.4	1.3	0	49	0	27
Milano, Pepperidge Farm	1	3.6	1.0	3	63	0	30
molasses	1	2.0	0.9	0	71	0	100
oatmeal	1	3.2	0.6	0	80	0	100
oatmeal raisin	1	3.0	0.8	0	83	0	28
oatmeal, Pepperidge Farm	1 large	6.4	1.0	5	120	1	105
Orleans, Pepperidge Farm	1	1.8	<1.0	0	31	0	10
peanut butter	1	3.2	1.0	6	72	1	36
Rice Krispie bar	1	0.9	0.3	0	36	0	38
shortbread	1	2.3	0.4	2	42	0	36
SnackWell's							
bite size chocolate chip	6	1.0	<1.0	0	60	0	85
cinnamon graham snacks	9	0	0	0	50	0	50
creme sandwich cookies	1	1.0	<1.0	0	50	0	50
devil's food cookie cakes	1	0	0	0	60	0	40
oatmeal raisin	1	1.0	<1.0	0	60	0	65
Social Tea biscuit	1	0.6	0.1	NA	22	0	18
sugar	1	3.4	1.0	8	89	0	60
sugar wafers	2 small	2.1	0.5	0	53	0	30
vanilla-creme sandwich	1	3.1	1.3	0	69	0	75
vanilla wafers	3	1.8	0.7	6	51	0	30
cream puff w/ custard	1	14.6	3.7	60	245	0	112
Creamsicle	1 bar	3.1	NA	0	103	0	27

Item	Serving	Total Fat (g)	Saturated Fat (g)	Cholesterol (mg)	Calories	Fiber (g)	Sodium (mg)
cupcake							
choc. w/icing	1	5.5	2.1	22	159	1	110
yellow w/icing	1	6.0	2.3	23	160	1	108
custard, baked	1/2 cup	6.9	3.4	123	148	0	104
date bar	1 bar	3.1	1.2	2	93	1	49
Dreamsicle	1 bar	6.2	3.9	17	207	0	137
dumpling, fruit	1 piece	15.1	5.5	8	324	2	256
eclair							
w/choc. icing & custard	1 small	15.4	5.7	115	316	0	147
w/choc. icing &							
whipped cream	1 small	25.7	11.3	NA	296	0	139
frosting/icing							
choc.	3 T	5.3	2.7	6	148	0	50
cream cheese	3 T	6.8	2.6	11	170	0	43
"light" varieties,							
ready-to-spread	1/12 tub	2.0	1.0	0	130	0	60
ready-to-spread	1/12 tub	6.9	2.5	4	169	0	30
seven-minute	3 T	0	0	0	135	0	25
vanilla or lemon	3 T	4.0	1.9	6	140	0	80
fruit ice, Italian	1/2 cup	0	0	0	123	0	0
fruitcake	1 piece	6.2	1.4	11	154	1	37
Fudgesicle	1 bar	0.4	0.2	3	196	1	248
gelatin							
low-cal.	1/2 cup	0	0	0	8	0	4
regular, sweetened	1/2 cup	0	0	0	70	0	50
granola bar	1 bar	6.8	1.5	0	141	1	79
Hostess							
cupcake	1	7.4	3.7	3	206	1	250
cupcake lights	1	2.0	<1.0	0	130	0	190
Ding Dong	1	8.7	4.0	6	170	0	130
fruit snack pie	1	20.2	6.9	12	403	2	449
Ho Ho	1	6.8	2.8	8	133	1	70

Item	Serving	Total Fat (g)	Saturated Fat (g)	Cholesterol (mg)	Calories	Fiber (g)	Sodium (mg)
Hostess *(cont.)*							
honey bun	1	33.3	NA	30	572	2	675
light apple spice	1	1.0	<1.0	0	130	0	150
light crumb cake	1	1.0	<1.0	0	80	0	95
Snoball	1	4.0	2.0	2	150	0	170
Twinkie	1	3.8	0.8	8	144	0	181
Twinkie lights	1	2.0	<1.0	0	110	0	160
ice cream							
choc. (10% fat)	1/2 cup	7.2	4.5	30	134	1	58
choc. (16% fat)	1/2 cup	11.9	7.4	44	174	0	54
dietetic, sugar-free	1/2 cup	7.0	4.4	27	134	0	48
French vanilla soft serve	1/2 cup	11.5	6.8	76	189	0	76
Simple Pleasures							
(simpless)	1/2 cup	0.5	0	10	120	0	65
strawberry (10% fat)	1/2 cup	6.0	4.0	28	128	0	55
vanilla (10% fat)	1/2 cup	7.2	4.5	30	134	0	58
vanilla (16% fat)	1/2 cup	11.9	7.4	44	175	0	54
Weight Watchers	1/2 cup	0.8	0.5	2	81	0	57
ice cream bar							
choc. coated	1 bar	11.5	10.0	23	178	0	28
toffee krunch	1 bar	10.2	7.0	9	149	1	52
ice cream cake roll	1 slice	6.9	4.0	52	159	0	88
ice cream cone							
(cone only)	1 medium	0.3	0.1	0	45	0	26
ice cream drumstick	1	10.0	4.1	14	188	1	58
ice cream sandwich	1	6.2	3.6	12	169	0	53
ice milk							
choc.	1/2 cup	3.1	1.8	9	91	0	52
soft serve, all flavors	1/2 cup	2.3	1.4	7	112	0	82
strawberry	1/2 cup	2.5	1.2	7	106	0	60
vanilla	1/2 cup	2.8	1.5	8	92	0	60
ladyfinger	1	2.0	0.5	80	79	0	15

Item	Serving	Total Fat (g)	Saturated Fat (g)	Cholesterol (mg)	Calories	Fiber (g)	Sodium (mg)
lemon bars	1 bar	3.2	0.7	13	70	0	49
Little Debbie							
devil square	1 square	5.2	NA	NA	131	0	75
Dutch apple bar	2 oz.	5.3	NA	NA	207	0	70
fudge krispie	2 oz.	7.1	NA	NA	256	1	70
oatmeal cremes	2 pieces	12.6	NA	NA	332	1	250
peanut-butter bar	2 bars	13.5	NA	NA	265	1	200
mousse, choc.	1/2 cup	15.5	8.7	124	189	1	37
napoleon	1 piece	5.3	2.6	10	85	0	35
pie							
apple	1/8 pie	16.9	2.3	3	347	3	195
banana cream or							
custard	1/8 pie	14.0	10.0	35	353	1	300
blueberry	1/8 pie	17.3	4.0	0	387	3	350
Boston cream pie	1/8 pie	8.4	2.8	20	260	1	225
cherry	1/8 pie	18.1	5.0	0	418	2	150
choc. cream	1/8 pie	13.0	4.5	15	311	3	427
choc. meringue,							
traditional	1/8 pie	18.0	6.5	NA	378	1	325
coconut cream or custard	1/8 pie	19.0	7.0	80	365	1	300
key lime	1/8 pie	19.0	6.8	10	388	1	290
lemon chiffon	1/8 pie	13.5	3.7	NA	335	1	300
lemon meringue,							
traditional	1/8 pie	13.1	5.1	8	350	1	260
mincemeat	1/8 pie	18.4	5.0	0	434	3	400
peach	1/8 pie	17.7	4.6	3	421	3	425
pecan	1/8 pie	23.0	3.5	100	510	2	250
pumpkin	1/8 pie	16.8	5.7	109	367	5	338
raisin	1/8 pie	12.9	3.1	0	325	1	336
rhubarb	1/8 pie	17.1	4.5	2	405	3	400
strawberry	1/8 pie	9.1	4.5	2	228	1	250
sweet potato	1/8 pie	18.2	6.0	70	342	2	300

Item	Serving	Total Fat (g)	Saturated Fat (g)	Cholesterol (mg)	Calories	Fiber (g)	Sodium (mg)
pie tart, fruit filled	1	18.7	6.2	23	362	2	NA
Popsicle	1 bar	0	0	0	96	0	0
pudding							
any flavor except choc.	1/2 cup	5.5	2.9	70	168	0	142
bread	1/2 cup	8.1	3.2	78	219	1	286
choc. w/whole milk	1/2 cup	8.6	4.9	47	247	1	140
choc., D-Zerta	1/2 cup	0.5	0.3	2	65	0	68
from mix w/skim milk	1/2 cup	0	0	0	124	0	125
noodle	1/2 cup	5.3	1.1	72	141	0	158
rice	1/2 cup	5.7	2.0	98	181	0	103
tapioca	1/2 cup	4.6	2.2	82	126	0	150
pudding pop, frzn	1 bar	2.0	1.0	2	75	0	80
sherbet	1/2 cup	1.8	1.2	7	135	0	44
sopaipilla	1 piece	6.0	0.8	0	88	0	68
soufflé, choc	1/2 cup	3.9	1.4	42	63	0	31
strudel, fruit	1/2 cup	1.2	0.1	2	47	1	12
Tasty Kake							
butterscotch Krimpet	1	2.1	0.9	7	118	0	94
choc. junior	1	12.2	3.5	4	306	1	298
coconut cream	1	31.2	10.2	39	482	1	286
fruit pie	1	14.3	5.1	48	362	2	370
jelly Krimpet	1	1.3	0.3	3	96	0	88
light creme-filled							
cupcakes	1	1.4	0.5	0	100	0	115
toppings							
butterscotch/caramel	3 T	0.1	0	0	156	0	109
cherry	3 T	0.1	0	0	147	0	10
choc. fudge	2 T	3.8	2.5	0	97	1	36
choc. syrup, Hershey	2 T	0.4	0.2	0	73	1	36
custard sauce, hmde	3 T	2.9	1.0	59	64	0	18
lemon sauce, hmde	3 T	2.1	0.4	10	100	0	20
marshmallow creme	3 T	0	0	0	158	0	17

Item	Serving	Total Fat (g)	Saturated Fat (g)	Cholesterol (mg)	Calories	Fiber (g)	Sodium (mg)
toppings *(cont.)*							
milk choc. fudge	2 T	5.0	2.9	NA	124	0	33
pecans in syrup	3 T	2.8	1.1	0	168	0	40
pineapple	3 T	0.2	0	0	146	0	20
raisin sauce, hmde	3 T	3.0	0.8	0	126	0	18
strawberry	3 T	0.1	0	0	139	0	10
whipped topping							
aerosol	1/4 cup	3.9	1.4	NA	46	0	3
from mix	1/4 cup	2.0	1.2	4	32	0	12
frzn, tub	1/4 cup	4.8	3.6	0	59	0	4
"lite"	1 T	<1.0	NA	NA	8	0	0
whipping cream							
heavy, fluid	1 T	5.6	3.5	21	52	0	6
light, fluid	1 T	4.6	2.9	17	44	0	5
trifle	1/2 cup	19.5	9.1	88	289	1	81
turnover, fruit filled	1	19.3	5.4	2	226	1	141
yogurt, frozen							
low fat	1/2 cup	3.0	2.0	10	115	0	55
nonfat	1/2 cup	0.2	0	0	81	0	39
EGGS							
boiled-poached	1	5.6	1.6	213	79	0	69
fried w/ 1/2 t fat	1 large	7.8	2.9	246	104	0	144
omelet							
2 oz. cheese,							
3 egg	1	37.0	12.3	480	510	0	838
plain, 3 egg	1	21.3	5.2	430	271	0	330
Spanish, 2 egg	1	18.0	5.9	375	250	1	225
scrambled w/milk	1 large	8.0	2.8	248	99	0	155
substitute, frzn	1/4 cup	0	0	0	30	0	80
white	1 large	0	0	0	16	0	50
yolk	1 large	5.6	1.6	213	63	0	8

Item	Serving	Total Fat (g)	Saturated Fat (g)	Cholesterol (mg)	Calories	Fiber (g)	Sodium (mg)
FAST FOOD/RESTAURANTS (all listings are for standard servings for the given establishment unless otherwise noted)							
Arby's							
baked potato deluxe	1	36.4	18.1	58	621	NA	605
beef 'n' cheddar sandwich	1	26.8	7.6	52	508	NA	1166
chicken breast sandwich	1	22.5	3.0	45	445	NA	958
curly fries	1 order	17.7	7.4	0	337	NA	167
french fries	1 order	13.2	3.0	0	246	NA	114
ham & cheese sandwich	1	14.2	5.1	55	355	NA	1400
jamocha shake	1	10.5	2.5	35	368	NA	262
junior roast-beef sandwich	1	10.8	4.1	22	233	NA	519
light roast beef deluxe	1	10.0	3.5	42	294	NA	826
light roast chicken deluxe	1	7.0	1.7	33	276	NA	777
light roast turkey deluxe	1	6.0	1.6	33	260	NA	1262
potato cakes	1 order	12.0	2.2	0	204	NA	397
roast-beef sandwich	1 regular	18.2	7.0	43	383	NA	936
roast-chicken club	1	27.0	6.9	46	503	NA	1143
roast chicken salad	1	7.2	3.3	43	204	NA	508
sausage biscuit	1	31.9	9.4	60	460	NA	1000
super roast-beef sandwich	1	28.3	7.6	43	552	NA	1174
Burger King							
apple pie	1	14.0	4.0	4	311	NA	412
bacon double cheeseburger	1	30.0	14.0	108	507	NA	809
bacon double cheeseburger deluxe	1	39.0	16.0	111	592	NA	804
BK Broiler chicken sandwich	1	8.0	2.0	45	267	NA	728

Item	Serving	Total Fat (g)	Saturated Fat (g)	Cholesterol (mg)	Calories	Fiber (g)	Sodium (mg)
Burger King (cont.)							
cheeseburger	1	15.0	7.0	50	318	NA	661
cheeseburger, deluxe	1	23.0	8.0	56	390	NA	652
cheeseburger, double	1	27.0	13.0	100	483	NA	851
chef salad	1	9.0	4.0	103	178	NA	568
cherry pie	1	13.0	4.0	4	311	NA	412
chicken sandwich	1	40.0	9.0	60	685	NA	1417
Chicken Tenders	1 order	13.0	3.0	38	236	NA	541
chunky chicken salad	1	4.0	1.0	49	142	NA	443
Croissan'wich w/bacon, egg, & cheese	1	23.0	8.0	230	353	NA	780
Croissan'wich w/ham, egg, & cheese	1	22.0	7.0	236	351	NA	1373
Croissan'wich w/sausage, egg, & cheese	1	40.0	14.0	258	534	NA	985
french fries, medium	1 order	20.0	10.0	21	341	NA	241
french toast sticks	1 order	32.0	8.0	52	538	NA	537
garden salad w/o dressing	1	5.0	3.0	15	95	NA	125
hamburger	1	11.0	4.0	37	272	NA	505
hamburger, deluxe	1	19.0	6.0	43	344	NA	496
mini muffins, blueberry	1 order	14.0	3.0	72	292	NA	244
Ocean Catch fish fillet	1	33.0	8.0	45	479	NA	736
onion rings, regular	1 order	19.0	5.0	0	339	NA	628
shakes							
choc.	1	10.0	6.0	31	326	NA	198
strawberry	1	10.0	6.0	33	394	NA	230
vanilla	1	10.0	6.0	33	334	NA	213
side salad							
w/diet dressing	1	0	0	0	42	NA	750
w/regular dressing	1	22.0	3.0	10	332	NA	400
Whopper	1	36.0	12.0	90	614	NA	865
Whopper w/cheese	1	44.0	16.0	115	706	NA	1177

Item	Serving	Total Fat (g)	Saturated Fat (g)	Cholesterol (mg)	Calories	Fiber (g)	Sodium (mg)
Burger King *(cont.)*							
Whopper, double beef	1	53.0	19.0	169	844	NA	933
Whopper, double beef w/cheese	1	61.0	24.0	194	935	NA	1245
Chick-Fil-A							
chargrilled chicken garden salad (w/Lite Italian dressing)	1	3.1	NA	NA	148	NA	NA
chargrilled chicken sandwich	1	4.8	NA	NA	258	NA	NA
chicken nuggets	8	15.0	NA	NA	287	NA	NA
Grilled 'n Lites	2 skewers	1.8	NA	NA	97	NA	NA
original chicken sandwich	1	8.5	NA	NA	360	NA	NA
Dairy Queen							
banana split	1	11.0	8.0	30	510	NA	250
Blizzard, strawberry	1 regular	16.0	11.0	50	570	NA	230
breaded chicken fillet sandwich	1	20.0	4.0	55	430	NA	760
breaded chicken fillet sandwich w/ cheese	1	25.0	7.0	70	480	NA	980
Breeze, strawberry	1 regular	1.0	<1.0	5	420	NA	170
Buster bar	1	29.0	9.0	15	450	NA	220
cheese dog	1	21.0	9.0	35	330	NA	920
cheeseburger	1	18.0	9.0	60	365	NA	800
cheeseburger, double	1	34.0	18.0	120	570	NA	1070
chili dog	1	19.0	7.0	30	330	NA	720
choc. sundae, regular	1	7.0	5.0	20	300	NA	140
Dilly bar	1	13.0	6.0	10	210	NA	50
DQ Homestyle Ultimate burger	1	47.0	21.0	140	700	NA	1100
DQ Sandwich, frozen treat	1	4.0	2.0	5	140	NA	135

Item	Serving	Total Fat (g)	Saturated Fat (g)	Cholesterol (mg)	Calories	Fiber (g)	Sodium (mg)
Dairy Queen *(cont.)*							
fish fillet sandwich	1	16.0	3.0	50	400	NA	630
fish fillet sandwich							
w/cheese	1	21.0	6.0	60	440	NA	850
french fries							
large	1 order	18.0	4.0	0	390	NA	200
regular	1 order	14.0	3.0	0	300	NA	160
small	1 order	10.0	2.0	0	210	NA	115
garden salad,							
plain	1	13.0	7.0	185	200	NA	240
grilled chicken fillet							
sandwich	1	8.0	2.0	50	300	NA	800
hamburger	1	13.0	6.0	45	310	NA	580
hamburger, double	1	25.0	12.0	95	470	NA	630
hot dog	1	16.0	6.0	25	280	NA	700
hot fudge brownie delight	1	29.0	14.0	35	710	NA	340
ice cream cone, regular							
choc.	1	7.0	5.0	20	230	NA	115
choc. dipped	1	16.0	8.0	20	330	NA	100
vanilla	1	7.0	5.0	20	230	NA	95
yogurt	1	<1.0	<1.0	<5	180	NA	80
onion rings	1 order	12.0	3.0	0	240	NA	135
Peanut Buster parfait	1	32.0	10.0	30	710	NA	410
shake, regular							
choc.	1	14.0	8.0	45	540	NA	210
vanilla	1	14.0	8.0	45	520	NA	230
yogurt strawberry							
sundae	1 regular	<1.0	<1.0	<5	200	NA	80
Dominos							
cheese pizza 12"	2 slices	10.0	5.0	20	360	NA	1000
deluxe pizza 12"	2 slices	23.0	10.5	50	540	NA	1760
extravaganza pizza 12"	2 slices	24.0	11.5	55	510	NA	1680

Item	Serving	Total Fat (g)	Saturated Fat (g)	Cholesterol (mg)	Calories	Fiber (g)	Sodium (mg)
Dominos *(cont.)*							
pepperoni pizza 12"	2 slices	15.0	7.5	35	410	NA	1190
pepperoni/sausage/							
mushroom pizza 12"	2 slices	20.0	9.0	50	460	NA	1410
sausage pizza 12"	2 slices	16.5	7.5	40	430	NA	1270
vegi feast pizza 12"	2 slices	13.0	6.5	25	390	NA	1090
Godfather's Pizza							
cheese pizza, large	1/10 pizza	7.0	NA	16	228	NA	464
combo pizza, large	1/10 pizza	19.0	NA	36	437	NA	1019
Hardee's							
apple turnover	1	12.0	4.0	0	268	NA	245
bacon biscuit	1	21.0	4.0	89	360	NA	950
bacon cheeseburger	1	39.0	16.0	80	610	NA	1030
bacon/egg/cheese/bagel	1	16.0	NA	175	375	NA	865
bagel, plain	1	3.0	NA	10	200	NA	350
Big Cookie Treat	1	13.0	4.0	5	250	NA	239
Big Country Breakfast							
w/bacon	1	40.0	10.0	305	660	NA	1540
w/ham	1	33.0	7.0	325	620	NA	1780
w/sausage	1	57.0	16.0	340	850	NA	1980
Big Deluxe burger	1	30.0	12.0	70	500	NA	760
biscuit 'n' gravy	1	24.0	6.0	15	440	NA	1250
blueberry muffin	1	17.0	4.0	65	400	NA	310
cheeseburger	1	14.0	6.0	40	300	NA	740
cheeseburger, 1/4 lb.	1	29.0	14.0	70	510	NA	1060
chef salad	1	13.0	8.0	44	214	NA	910
chicken fillet	1	13.0	2.0	55	370	NA	1060
chicken stix	6 pieces	9.0	2.0	35	210	NA	678
cinnamon 'n' raisin							
biscuit	1	17.0	5.0	0	315	NA	515
fisherman's fillet	1	21.0	5.0	65	470	NA	1140
french fries, regular	1 order	11.0	2.0	0	230	NA	85

Item	Serving	Total Fat (g)	Saturated Fat (g)	Cholesterol (mg)	Calories	Fiber (g)	Sodium (mg)
Hardee's *(cont.)*							
fried chicken breast	1	19.0	7.0	104	340	NA	659
Frisco breakfast sandwich	1	20.0	7.0	205	430	NA	1110
Frisco burger	1	47.0	17.0	80	730	NA	1110
Frisco chicken	1	41.0	10.0	100	680	NA	1680
Frisco club	1	42.0	12.0	90	670	NA	1870
garden salad	1	12.0	7.0	34	184	NA	250
grilled chicken breast sandwich	1	9.0	1.0	60	310	NA	890
grilled chicken salad	1	4.0	1.0	60	120	NA	520
ham sub	1	7.0	4.0	45	370	NA	1400
hamburger	1	10.0	4.0	30	260	NA	510
Hash Rounds	1 order	14.0	3.0	0	230	NA	560
hot dog	1	16.0	4.0	30	290	NA	760
mushroom 'n' Swiss burger	1	28.0	13.0	70	490	NA	940
pancakes	1 order	2.0	1.0	15	280	NA	890
rise 'n' shine biscuit	1	18.0	3.0	0	320	NA	740
roast-beef sandwich	1	11.0	4.0	40	280	NA	870
sausage biscuit	1	28.0	7.0	25	440	NA	1100
side salad	1	<1.0	0	0	19	NA	14
steak biscuit	1	29.0	7.0	30	500	NA	1320
turkey club sandwich	1	16.0	4.0	70	390	NA	1280
turkey sub	1	7.0	4.0	65	390	NA	1420
Jack in the Box							
apple turnover	1	19.0	4.4	0	354	1	479
Breakfast Jack sandwich	1	13.0	5.2	203	301	0	871
cheeseburger	1	14.0	5.7	41	315	0	746
cheeseburger, Jumbo Jack	1	40.0	14.0	102	677	1	1090
cheeseburger, Ultimate	1	69.0	26.4	127	942	NA	1176
chef salad	1	18.0	8.4	142	325	NA	900
chicken fajita pita	1	8.0	2.9	34	292	NA	703

Item	Serving	Total Fat (g)	Saturated Fat (g)	Cholesterol (mg)	Calories	Fiber (g)	Sodium (mg)
Jack in the Box (cont.)							
chicken strips	4 pieces	13.0	3.1	52	285	NA	695
chicken supreme sandwich	1	39.0	10.0	85	641	NA	1470
chicken wings	6 pieces	44.0	10.7	181	846	NA	1710
fish supreme sandwich	1	27.0	6.1	55	510	NA	1040
french fries, regular	1 order	17.0	4.0	0	351	1	194
grilled chicken fillet sandwich	1	19.0	4.7	65	431	NA	1070
grilled sourdough burger	1	50.0	15.9	109	712	NA	1140
hamburger	1	11.0	4.1	26	267	0	555
hamburger, Jumbo Jack	1	34.0	11.0	70	584	1	733
onion rings	1 order	23.0	5.5	0	380	0	451
pancake platter	1	22.0	8.6	99	612	NA	888
scrambled egg platter	1	32.0	8.7	378	559	NA	1060
shake							
choc.	1	7.0	4.3	25	330	0	270
vanilla	1	6.0	3.6	25	320	0	230
sourdough breakfast sandwich	1	20.0	7.1	236	381	NA	1120
supreme crescent	1	40.0	13.2	178	547	NA	1053
taco salad	1	31.0	13.4	92	503	NA	1600
Kentucky Fried chicken (KFC)							
breast, extra crispy	1	23.0	6.0	80	365	0	640
breast, hot & spicy	1	26.0	7.0	84	382	0	905
breast, original recipe	1	14.0	4.0	92	260	0	609
Chicken Little sandwich	1	10.0	2.0	18	169	1	331
chicken nuggets	6 nuggets	18.0	4.0	66	284	0	865
coleslaw	1 order	6.0	1.0	4	114	0	177
Colonel's chicken sandwich	1	27.0	6.0	47	482	1	1060

Item	Serving	Total Fat (g)	Saturated Fat (g)	Cholesterol (mg)	Calories	Fiber (g)	Sodium (mg)
Kentucky Fried Chicken *(cont.)*							
corn on the cob	1 ear	2.0	1.0	0	90	1	11
crispy fries	1 order	17.0	4.0	3	294	1	761
drumstick, extra crispy	1	14.0	3.0	72	205	0	292
drumstick, hot & spicy	1	14.0	3.0	75	207	0	406
drumstick, original recipe	1	9.0	2.0	75	152	0	269
french fries	1 order	12.0	3.0	2	244	1	139
Hot Wings	6	33.0	8.0	150	471	0	1230
mashed potatoes & gravy	1 order	2.0	0.0	<1	71	0	339
Rotisserie Gold Chicken							
Dark Quarter (as served)	1	23.7	6.6	163	333	0	980
Dark Quarter (skin removed)	1	12.2	3.5	128	217	0	772
White Quarter (as served)	1	18.7	5.4	157	335	0	1104
White Quarter (skin removed)	1	5.9	1.7	97	199	0	667
thigh, extra crispy	1	31.0	8.0	112	414	0	580
thigh, original recipe	1	21.0	5.0	112	287	0	591
wing, extra crispy	1	17.0	4.0	63	231	0	319
wing, original recipe	1	11.0	3.0	59	172	0	383
Long John Silver's							
baked chicken dinner	1	15.0	3.2	75	550	NA	1670
batter-dipped fish	1 piece	11.0	2.7	30	180	NA	490
batter-dipped shrimp	1 piece	2.0	0.5	10	30	NA	80
Chicken Plank	1 piece	6.0	1.6	15	120	NA	400
Chicken Planks (dinner)	3 pieces	44.0	9.5	55	890	NA	2000
chicken sandwich	1	8.0	2.1	15	280	NA	790
clam dinner	1	52.0	10.9	75	990	NA	1830
coleslaw	1/2 cup	6.0	1.0	15	140	NA	260

Item	Serving	Total Fat (g)	Saturated Fat (g)	Cholesterol (mg)	Calories	Fiber (g)	Sodium (mg)
Long John Silver's *(cont.)*							
corn cobbette	1	8.0	NA	0	140	NA	10
fish & fries	2 piece	37.0	7.9	60	610	NA	1480
Fish & More dinner	2 piece	48.0	10.1	75	890	NA	1790
fish sandwich							
(w/out sauce)	1	13.0	3.2	30	340	NA	890
fish w/lemon crumb	1 dinner	12.0	2.1	125	570	NA	1470
french fries	1 order	15.0	2.5	0	250	NA	500
hush puppies	3	6.0	1.2	10	210	NA	75
Light Portion fish	1 dinner	5.0	0.8	75	270	NA	680
Ocean chef salad	1	1.0	0.4	40	110	NA	730
seafood chowder	7 oz.	6.0	1.8	20	140	NA	590
seafood gumbo	7 oz.	8.0	2.1	25	120	NA	740
seafood salad	1	31.0	5.1	55	380	NA	980
shrimp dinner	1	47.0	9.7	100	840	NA	1630
McDonald's							
apple bran muffin	1	0	0	0	180	NA	200
bacon bits	1 pkg.	1.2	0.5	1	16	0	95
Big Mac	1	26.0	9.0	100	500	1	890
biscuit w/bacon, egg,							
& cheese	1	26.4	8.2	253	440	1	1215
biscuit w/sausage	1	28.0	8.0	44	420	1	1040
biscuit w/sausage							
& egg	1	33.0	10.0	260	505	1	1210
biscuit w/spread	1	12.7	3.4	1	260	1	730
breakfast burrito	1	17.0	4.0	135	280	1	580
cheeseburger	1	13.8	5.2	53	305	0	725
chef salad w/o dressing	1	9.0	4.0	111	170	1	400
chicken fajitas	1	8.0	2.0	35	185	1	310
Chicken McNuggets	6 pieces	15.0	3.5	55	270	0	580
chunky chicken salad							
w/o dressing	1	4.0	1.0	78	150	1	230

Item	Serving	Total Fat (g)	Saturated Fat (g)	Cholesterol (mg)	Calories	Fiber (g)	Sodium (mg)
McDonald's *(cont.)*							
cookies							
choc. chip	1 box	15.0	4.0	4	330	0	280
McDonaldland	1 box	9.2	1.0	0	290	0	300
croutons	1 pkg.	2.2	0.5	0	50	NA	140
Danish, all varieties	1	18.0	4.5	35	420	0	400
Egg McMuffin	1	11.2	3.8	226	290	0	71
English muffin w/spread	1	4.0	1.0	0	170	1	285
Filet-O-Fish	1	18.0	4.0	50	370	0	730
french fries							
small	1 order	12.0	2.5	0	220	1	110
medium	1 order	17.1	3.5	0	320	1	150
large	1 order	21.6	5.0	0	400	1	200
frozen yogurt cone	1	0.8	0.4	3	105	0	80
garden salad							
w/o dressing	1	2.0	0.6	65	50	1	70
hamburger	1	9.0	3.0	37	255	0	490
hash browns	1 order	7.3	1.0	0	130	0	330
hotcakes w/margarine							
& syrup	1	12.0	2.0	8	440	0	685
McChicken sandwich	1	20.0	4.0	50	415	0	830
McLean Deluxe	1	10.0	4.0	60	320	NA	670
McLean w/cheese	1	14.0	5.0	75	370	NA	890
pie, apple	1	14.8	4.8	6	260	0	240
Quarter Pounder	1	20.7	8.1	86	410	1	645
Quarter Pounder							
w/cheese	1	28.0	11.2	118	520	1	1110
sausage, pork	1	15.0	5.0	43	160	0	310
Sausage McMuffin	1	20.0	7.0	57	345	1	770
Sausage McMuffin							
w/egg	1	25.0	8.0	270	430	1	920
scrambled eggs (2)	1 order	9.8	3.3	425	140	0	290

Item	Serving	Total Fat (g)	Saturated Fat (g)	Cholesterol (mg)	Calories	Fiber (g)	Sodium (mg)
McDonald's *(cont.)*							
shake							
choc.	1	1.7	0.8	10	320	0	240
strawberry	1	1.3	0.6	10	320	0	170
vanilla	1	1.3	0.6	10	290	0	170
side salad w/o dressing	1	1.0	0.3	33	30	1	35
sundae							
caramel	1	2.8	1.5	13	270	0	180
hot fudge	1	3.2	2.4	6	240	0	170
strawberry	1	1.1	0.6	5	210	0	95
Pizza Hut							
Hand-Tossed pizza							
cheese, medium	2 slices	20.0	13.6	55	518	NA	1276
pepperoni, medium	2 slices	23.0	12.9	50	500	NA	1267
supreme, medium	2 slices	26.0	13.8	55	540	NA	1470
Pan pizza							
cheese, medium	2 slices	18.0	9.0	34	492	NA	940
pepperoni, medium	2 slices	22.0	9.2	42	540	NA	1127
supreme, medium	2 slices	30.0	13.8	48	589	NA	1363
Thin 'n' Crispy pizza							
cheese, medium	2 slices	17.0	10.4	33	398	NA	867
pepperoni, medium	2 slices	20.0	10.6	46	413	NA	986
supreme, medium	2 slices	22.0	11.0	42	459	NA	1328
Shoney's Restaurants							
All American burger	1	32.6	NA	86	501	1	597
baked fish, light	1	1.4	NA	83	170	0	1641
baked potato (10 oz.)	1	0.3	NA	0	264	7	16
charbroiled chicken	1	6.1	NA	85	198	0	491
charbroiled chicken							
sandwich	1	17.0	NA	90	451	1	1002
charbroiled shrimp	1 order	3.0	NA	162	138	0	170
chicken fillet sandwich	1	21.2	NA	51	464	1	585

Item	Serving	Total Fat (g)	Saturated Fat (g)	Cholesterol (mg)	Calories	Fiber (g)	Sodium (mg)
Shoney's Restaurants *(cont.)*							
chicken tenders	1 order	20.4	NA	64	388	0	239
country-fried steak	1	27.2	NA	27	449	1	1177
french fries (3 oz.)	1 order	7.5	NA	0	189	3	26
french toast sticks	1 order	2.9	NA	0	69	0	157
garden salad, typical (9 oz. fresh veg./ low-cal. dress.)	1	0.6	NA	0	63	5	601
Grecian bread	1	2.2	NA	0	80	0	94
half-o-pound dinner	1	34.4	NA	123	435	0	280
Hawaiian chicken	1	6.2	NA	85	221	0	492
hot fudge sundae	1	22.0	NA	60	451	0	226
lasagna	1	9.8	NA	26	297	3	870
liver and onions	1	22.9	NA	529	411	1	321
onion rings	each	3.1	NA	2	52	0	43
pancakes	1	0.1	NA	0	41	0	238
rice (3.5 oz.)	1	3.7	NA	1	137	0	765
shrimper's feast	1	22.2	NA	125	383	0	216
sirloin	6 oz.	24.5	NA	64	357	0	160
Slim Jim	1	23.9	NA	57	484	1	1620
soups, Lightside, average	1	1.7	NA	4	73	1	503
spaghetti dinner	1	16.3	NA	55	496	2	387
strawberry pie	1 slice	16.7	NA	0	332	2	247
Taco Bell							
burrito, bean	1	14.0	4.0	9	381	1	1148
burrito, beef	1	21.0	8.0	59	43	NA	1311
burrito, chicken	1	12.0	NA	52	334	NA	880
burrito, combo	1	16.0	10.0	33	407	NA	1136
burrito, Supreme	1	22.0	9.0	35	440	NA	1181
chilito	1	18.0	NA	47	383	NA	893
cinnamon twists	1 order	8.0	3.0	0	171	NA	234

Item	Serving	Total Fat (g)	Saturated Fat (g)	Cholesterol (mg)	Calories	Fiber (g)	Sodium (mg)
Taco Bell *(cont.)*							
Mexican pizza	1	37.0	NA	52	575	NA	1031
MexiMelt, beef	1	15.0	NA	38	266	NA	689
MexiMelt, chicken	1	15.0	NA	48	257	NA	779
nachos	1 order	18.0	NA	9	346	NA	399
nachos, Supreme	1 order	27.0	NA	18	367	NA	471
pintos 'n cheese	1 order	9.0	4.0	16	190	NA	642
soft taco	1	12.0	NA	32	225	NA	554
soft taco, chicken	1	10.0	NA	52	213	NA	615
soft taco, Supreme	1	16.0	NA	32	272	NA	554
taco	1	11.0	4.0	32	183	1	274
taco salad	1	61.0	NA	80	905	NA	910
tostada	1	11.0	5.0	18	243	NA	596
Wendy's							
baked potato, plain	1	0	0	0	300	4	20
baked potato, w/cheese	1	24.0	8.0	30	550	4	640
Big Classic	1	23.0	7.0	75	480	NA	850
breaded chicken sandwich	1	20.0	4.0	60	450	1	740
breadstick	1	3.0	1.0	5	130	NA	250
Caesar side salad	1	6.0	1.0	10	160	NA	700
cheeseburger, single	1	21.0	9.5	85	420	1	770
cheeseburger, junior	1	13.0	5.0	45	320	NA	760
chicken club sandwich	1	25.0	6.0	75	520	NA	980
chili con carne	1 small	6.0	4.0	15	370	2	35
country fried steak sandwich	1	26.0	7.0	35	460	NA	880
crispy chicken nuggets (6)	1	20.0	4.5	50	280	NA	600
deluxe garden salad	1	5.0	1.0	0	110	NA	300
fish fillet sandwich	1	25.0	5.0	55	460	NA	780

Item	Serving	Total Fat (g)	Saturated Fat (g)	Cholesterol (mg)	Calories	Fiber (g)	Sodium (mg)
Wendy's *(cont.)*							
french fries (small)	1 order	12.0	2.5	0	240	NA	145
Frosty, choc., small	1	10.0	5.0	40	340	0	200
grilled chicken salad	1	8.0	1.0	55	200	NA	690
grilled chicken							
sandwich	1	7.0	1.0	60	290	1	670
hamburger, single	1	15.0	6.0	70	350	1	510
hamburger, double	1	27.0	11.0	140	540	1	730
hamburger, junior	1	9.0	3.3	34	260	NA	590
taco salad	1	30.0	12.0	80	640	NA	960
FATS							
bacon fat	1 T	14.0	3.6	9	126	0	126
beef, separable fat	1 oz.	23.3	6.0	24	216	0	5
butter							
solid	1 t	4.1	2.3	11	36	0	26
solid	1 T	12.3	6.9	33	108	0	78
whipped	1 t	3.1	1.9	8	28	0	31
Butter Buds, liquid	2 T	0	NA	0	12	0	170
butter sprinkles	1/2 t	0	0	0	4	0	75
chicken fat, raw	1 T	12.8	3.8	11	115	0	0
cream							
light	1 T	2.9	1.8	10	29	0	6
medium (25% fat)	1 T	3.8	2.3	13	37	0	6
cream substitute							
liquid/frzn	1/2 fl. oz.	1.5	0.3	0	20	0	12
powdered	1 T	0.7	0.7	0	11	0	4
half & half	1 T	1.7	1.1	6	20	0	6
margarine							
liquid	1 t	4.0	0.6	0	35	0	37
reduced calorie, tub	1 t	2.0	0.3	0	18	0	46
solid (corn), stick	1 t	4.0	0.6	0	35	0	44

Item	Serving	Total Fat (g)	Saturated Fat (g)	Cholesterol (mg)	Calories	Fiber (g)	Sodium (mg)
mayonnaise							
fat-free	1 T	0	0	0	12	0	150
reduced calorie	1 T	4.5	0.6	3	44	0	96
regular (soybean)	1 T	11.0	1.6	8	99	0	78
no-stick spray (Pam, etc.)	2-sec spray	0.8	0.1	0	8	0	0
oil							
canola	1 T	14.0	1.3	0	120	0	0
corn	1 T	14.0	1.7	0	120	0	0
olive	1 T	14.0	1.8	0	119	0	0
safflower	1 T	14.0	1.2	0	120	0	0
soybean	1 T	14.0	2.0	0	120	0	0
pork							
backfat, raw	1 oz.	25.4	6.5	20	192	0	7
separable fat,							
cooked	1 oz.	23.4	7.8	26	216	0	9
pork fat (lard)	1 T	12.8	5.0	12	116	0	0
salt pork, raw	1 oz.	23.8	8.3	25	219	0	404
sandwich spread (Miracle							
Whip type	1 T	7.0	1.1	6	69	0	84
shortening, vegetable	1 T	12.0	3.1	0	106	0	0
sour cream							
cultured	1 T	2.5	1.6	5	26	0	6
fat-free	1 T	0	0	0	8	0	10
half & half, cultured	1 T	1.8	1.1	6	20	0	6
imitation	1 T	2.7	2.3	0	25	0	13
"lite"	1 T	1.0	0.5	3	20	0	18
reduced calorie	1 T	1.3	0.6	4	15	0	15
FISH (all baked/broiled w/o added fat unless otherwise noted)							
abalone, canned	3 1/2 oz.	0.3	0.1	97	80	0	298
anchovy, canned	3 fillets	1.2	0.2	12	21	0	370

Item	Serving	Total Fat (g)	Saturated Fat (g)	Cholesterol (mg)	Calories	Fiber (g)	Sodium (mg)
anchovy paste	1 t	0.8	NA	NA	14	0	NA
bass							
freshwater	3 1/2 oz.	2.6	0.7	60	104	0	60
saltwater, baked w/fat	3 1/2 oz.	19.4	NA	NA	287	0	168
saltwater, black	3 1/2 oz.	1.2	0.2	50	93	0	68
saltwater, striped	3 1/2 oz.	2.7	0.7	70	105	0	60
bluefish							
cooked	3 1/2 oz.	3.3	0.8	50	117	0	51
fried	3 1/2 oz.	12.8	2.7	59	205	0	78
buffalofish	3 1/2 oz.	4.2	0.8	72	150	0	34
butterfish							
gulf	3 1/2 oz.	2.9	0.7	60	95	0	80
northern	3 1/2 oz.	10.2	1.9	49	184	0	59
northern, fried	3 1/2 oz.	19.1	2.5	50	275	0	160
carp	3 1/2 oz.	5.8	1.2	72	138	0	54
catfish	3 1/2 oz.	3.1	0.7	60	103	0	50
catfish, breaded & fried	3 1/2 oz.	13.2	2.9	81	226	NA	278
caviar, sturgeon,							
granular	1 round t	1.5	0.4	47	26	0	150
clams							
canned, solids & liquid	1/2 cup	0.7	0.1	25	52	0	45
canned, solids only	3 oz.	2.5	0.2	57	126	0	95
meat only	5 large	0.9	0.1	42	80	0	70
soft, raw	4 large	1.9	0.1	29	63	0	47
cod							
canned	3 1/2 oz.	0.3	0.1	45	85	0	180
cooked	3 1/2 oz.	0.3	0.1	40	78	0	60
dried, salted	3 1/2 oz.	1.7	0.4	129	246	0	5973
crab							
canned	1/2 cup	2.1	0.2	76	86	0	283
deviled	3 1/2 oz.	9.9	3.5	40	188	0	450
fried	3 1/2 oz.	18.0	NA	NA	273	0	NA

Item	Serving	Total Fat (g)	Saturated Fat (g)	Cholesterol (mg)	Calories	Fiber (g)	Sodium (mg)
crab, Alaska king	3 1/2 oz.	1.5	NA	53	96	0	1062
crab cake	3 1/2 oz.	10.8	1.2	100	178	0	225
crappie, white	3 1/2 oz.	0.8	0.3	60	79	0	104
crayfish, freshwater	3 1/2 oz.	0.5	0.2	115	72	0	45
crooker							
Atlantic	3 1/2 oz.	3.2	1.0	60	133	0	50
white	3 1/2 oz.	0.8	0.3	60	84	0	104
cusk, steamed	3 1/2 oz.	0.7	0.2	NA	106	0	110
dolphinfish	3 1/2 oz.	0.7	0.2	72	85	0	86
eel, American							
cooked	3 1/2 oz.	18.3	4.2	74	260	0	82
smoked	3 1/2 oz.	23.6	4.9	60	281	0	679
eulachon (smelt)	3 1/2 oz.	6.2	1.3	49	118	0	59
fillets, frzn							
batter dipped	2 pieces	31.0	NA	NA	440	0	552
light & crispy	2 pieces	23.0	NA	NA	311	0	345
fish cakes, frzn,							
fried	3 1/2 oz.	14.0	3.9	102	242	2	567
flatfish	3 1/2 oz.	0.8	0.2	47	79	0	69
flounder/sole	3 1/2 oz.	0.5	0.2	30	68	0	56
gefilte fish	3 1/2 oz.	2.2	0.5	50	82	1	155
grouper	3 1/2 oz.	1.3	0.4	47	87	0	53
haddock							
cooked	3 1/2 oz.	0.6	0.1	50	79	0	58
fried	3 1/2 oz.	10.0	3.0	60	180	0	130
smoked/canned	3 1/2 oz.	0.4	0.1	68	103	0	655
halibut	3 1/2 oz.	1.2	0.5	30	100	0	50
herring							
canned or smoked	3 1/2 oz.	13.6	2.2	66	208	0	734
cooked	3 1/2 oz.	11.3	2.0	70	176	0	90
pickled	3 1/2 oz.	15.1	2.4	70	223	0	786
Jack mackerel	3 1/2 oz.	5.6	1.7	75	143	0	360

Item	Serving	Total Fat (g)	Saturated Fat (g)	Cholesterol (mg)	Calories	Fiber (g)	Sodium (mg)
kingfish	3 1/2 oz.	3.0	0.8	68	105	0	83
lake trout	3 1/2 oz.	19.9	4.2	74	241	0	82
lobster, northern							
broiled w/fat	12 oz.	24.0	NA	NA	308	0	NA
cooked	3 1/2 oz.	1.9	0.1	65	91	0	325
mackerel							
Atlantic	3 1/2 oz.	12.2	2.9	65	191	0	80
Pacific	3 1/2 oz.	7.3	2.2	50	159	0	80
muskekunge							
("muskie," "skie")	3 1/2 oz.	2.5	0.6	70	109	0	75
mussels							
canned	3 1/2 oz.	3.3	NA	NA	114	0	NA
meat only	3 1/2 oz.	2.2	0.7	30	95	0	250
ocean perch							
cooked	3 1/2 oz.	1.2	0.5	40	88	0	70
fried	3 1/2 oz.	13.3	NA	NA	227	0	NA
octopus	3 1/2 oz.	0.8	0.3	48	73	0	NA
oysters							
canned	3 1/2 oz.	2.2	0.8	54	76	0	100
fried	3 1/2 oz.	13.9	3.2	83	239	0	426
raw	5-8 medium	1.8	0.6	54	66	0	110
scalloped	6 medium	18.0	NA	NA	356	0	NA
perch, freshwater,							
yellow	3 1/2 oz.	0.9	0.4	80	91	0	58
pickerel	3 1/2 oz.	0.5	0.1	NA	84	0	NA
pike							
blue	3 1/2 oz.	0.9	0.5	75	90	0	45
northern	3 1/2 oz.	1.1	0.7	40	88	0	40
walleye	3 1/2 oz.	1.2	1.0	80	93	0	50
pollock, Atlantic	3 1/2 oz.	1.0	0.2	70	91	0	85
pompano	3 1/2 oz.	9.5	5.0	55	166	0	65
red snapper	3 1/2 oz.	1.9	0.5	35	93	0	60

Item	Serving	Total Fat (g)	Saturated Fat (g)	Cholesterol (mg)	Calories	Fiber (g)	Sodium (mg)
rockfish, oven steamed	3 1/2 oz.	2.5	0.8	40	107	0	70
roughy, orange	3 1/2 oz.	7.0	0.1	20	124	0	63
salmon							
Atlantic	3 1/2 oz.	6.3	0.9	55	141	0	43
broiled/baked	3 1/2 oz.	7.4	2.0	50	182	0	60
chinook, canned	3 1/2 oz.	14.0	2.0	60	210	0	800
pink, canned	3 1/2 oz.	5.1	1.3	54	118	0	471
smoked	3 1/2 oz.	9.3	1.0	35	176	0	900
sardines							
Atlantic, in soy oil	2 sardines	2.8	0.4	34	50	0	121
Pacific	3 1/2 oz.	8.6	2.5	50	160	0	310
scallops							
cooked	3 1/2 oz.	1.2	0.2	30	81	0	140
frzn, fried	3 1/2 oz.	10.5	2.3	55	194	0	417
steamed	3 1/2 oz.	1.4	0.2	40	112	0	260
sea bass, white	3 1/2 oz.	1.5	0.6	40	96	0	65
shrimp							
canned, dry pack	3 1/2 oz.	1.6	0.5	155	116	0	150
canned, wet pack	1/2 cup	0.8	0.3	125	87	0	1956
fried	3 1/2 oz.	10.8	0.9	120	225	0	186
raw or broiled	3 1/2 oz.	1.8	0.7	139	91	0	130
smelt, canned	4-5 medium	13.5	NA	NA	200	0	NA
sole, fillet	3 1/2 oz.	0.5	0.2	30	68	0	160
squid							
fried	3 oz.	6.4	NA	NA	149	0	NA
raw	3 oz.	1.2	0.4	261	110	0	49
surimi	3 1/2 oz.	0.9	0.2	30	98	0	142
sushi or sashimi	3 1/2 oz.	4.9	1.3	38	144	0	38
swordfish	3 1/2 oz.	4.0	1.1	43	118	0	96
trout							
brook	3 1/2 oz.	2.1	0.9	53	101	0	25
rainbow	3 1/2 oz.	11.4	1.2	96	195	0	46

Item	Serving	Total Fat (g)	Saturated Fat (g)	Cholesterol (mg)	Calories	Fiber (g)	Sodium (mg)
tuna							
albacore, raw	3 1/2 oz.	7.5	0.2	70	177	0	542
bluefin, raw	3 1/2 oz.	4.1	1.3	37	145	0	39
canned, light in oil	3 1/2 oz.	8.1	1.5	18	197	0	351
canned, light in water	3 1/2 oz.	0.8	0.2	30	115	0	336
canned, white in oil	3 1/2 oz.	8.0	1.6	31	185	0	393
canned, white in water	3 1/2 oz.	2.4	0.6	42	135	0	389
yellowfin, raw	3 1/2 oz.	3.0	0.5	57	133	0	41
white perch	3 1/2 oz.	3.9	0.7	65	114	0	45
whiting	3 1/2 oz.	1.7	0.4	83	114	0	130
yellowtail	3 1/2 oz.	5.4	0.9	75	138	0	46
FRUIT							
apple							
dried	1/2 cup	0.1	0	0	155	5	56
whole w/peel	1 medium	0.4	0.1	0	81	4	1
applesauce,							
unsweetened	1/2 cup	0.1	0	0	53	2	0
apricots							
dried	5 halves	0.3	0	0	83	6	3
fresh	3 medium	0.4	0	0	51	2	1
avocado							
California	1 (6 oz.)	30.0	4.5	0	306	4	21
Florida	1 (11 oz.)	27.0	5.3	0	339	4	14
banana	1 medium	0.6	0.2	0	105	2	1
banana chips	1/2 cup	15.5	13.4	0	239	4	3
blackberries							
fresh	1 cup	0.5	0	0	74	7	0
frzn, unsweetened	1 cup	0.7	0	0	97	7	0
blueberries							
fresh	1 cup	0.6	0	0	82	5	9
frzn, unsweetened	1 cup	0.7	0.2	0	80	4	1

Item	Serving	Total Fat (g)	Saturated Fat (g)	Cholesterol (mg)	Calories	Fiber (g)	Sodium (mg)
boysenberries, frzn							
unsweetened	1 cup	0.3	0	0	66	6	2
breadfruit, fresh	1/4 small	0.2	0	0	99	3	2
cantaloupe	1 cup	0.4	0	0	57	3	14
cherries							
maraschino	1/4 cup	0.1	0	0	56	1	2
sour, canned in heavy							
syrup	1/2 cup	0.4	0	0	116	1	9
sweet	1/2 cup	0.7	0.1	0	49	2	0
cranberries, fresh	1 cup	0.2	0	0	46	4	1
cranberry sauce	1/2 cup	0.2	0	0	209	1	40
cranberry-orange relish	1/2 cup	0.9	0	0	246	3	44
dates, whole, dried	1/2 cup	0.4	0	0	228	8	2
figs							
canned	3 figs	0.1	0	0	75	9	1
dried, uncooked	10 figs	1.0	0.4	0	477	16	20
fresh	1 medium	0.2	0	0	37	2	1
fruit cocktail, canned							
w/juice	1 cup	0.3	0	0	112	5	8
fruit roll-up	1	0	0	0	50	0	7
grapefruit	1/2 medium	0.1	0	0	39	1	0
grapes, Thompson							
seedless	1/2 cup	0.3	0	0	94	1	7
guava, fresh	1 medium	0.5	0.2	0	45	7	2
honeydew melon, fresh	1/4 small	0.3	0	0	33	1	12
kiwi, fresh	1 medium	0.3	0	0	46	2	4
kumquat, fresh	1 medium	0	0	0	12	1	1
lemon, fresh	1 medium	0.2	0	0	17	1	1
lime, fresh	1 medium	0.1	0	0	20	1	1
mandarin oranges, canned							
w/juice	1/2 cup	0.1	0	0	46	4	7
mango, fresh	1 medium	0.6	0.1	0	135	4	4

Item	Serving	Total Fat (g)	Saturated Fat (g)	Cholesterol (mg)	Calories	Fiber (g)	Sodium (mg)
melon balls, frzn	1 cup	0.4	0	0	55	2	53
mixed fruit							
dried	1/2 cup	0.5	0	0	243	6	18
frzn, sweetened	1 cup	0.5	0.2	0	245	2	8
mulberries, fresh	1 cup	0.6	0	0	61	3	14
nectarine, fresh	1 medium	0.6	0	0	67	2	0
orange							
naval, fresh	1 medium	0.2	0	0	65	4	1
Valencia, fresh	1 medium	0.4	0	0	59	4	0
papaya, fresh	1 medium	0.4	0.1	0	117	3	8
passionfruit, purple, fresh	1 medium	0.1	0	0	18	3	5
peach							
canned in heavy syrup	1 cup	0.3	0	0	190	4	16
canned in light syrup	1 cup	0.2	0	0	136	4	13
canned, water pack	1 cup	0.1	0	0	58	4	8
fresh	1 medium	0.1	0	0	37	1	0
frzn, sweetened	1 cup	0.3	0	0	235	4	16
pear							
canned in heavy syrup	1 cup	0.3	0	0	188	6	13
canned in light syrup	1 cup	0.1	0	0	144	6	13
fresh	1 medium	0.7	0	0	98	5	1
persimmon, fresh	1 medium	0.1	0	0	32	3	0
pineapple pieces							
canned, unsweetened	1 cup	0.2	0	0	150	2	4
fresh	1 cup	0.7	0	0	77	3	1
plantain, cooked, sliced	1 cup	0.3	0	0	179	1	8
plum							
canned in heavy syrup	1/2 cup	0.1	0	0	119	4	26
fresh	1 medium	0.6	0	0	36	3	0
pomegranate, fresh	1 medium	0.5	0	0	104	2	5
prickly pear, fresh	1 medium	0.5	0	0	42	3	6
prunes, dried, cooked	1/2 cup	0.2	0	0	113	10	2

Item	Serving	Total Fat (g)	Saturated Fat (g)	Cholesterol (mg)	Calories	Fiber (g)	Sodium (mg)
raisins							
dark seedless	1/4 cup	0.2	0.1	0	112	3	8
golden seedless	1/4 cup	0.2	0.1	0	113	3	4
raspberries							
fresh	1 cup	0.2	0	0	61	6	0
frzn, sweetened	1 cup	0.4	0	0	103	12	1
rhubarb, stewed,							
unsweetened	1 cup	0	0	0	12	6	5
star fruit/carambola	1 medium	0.4	0	0	42	2	3
strawberries							
fresh	1 cup	0.2	0	0	45	3	2
frzn, sweetened	1 cup	0.3	0	0	245	3	3
frzn, unsweetened	1 cup	0.2	0	0	52	3	8
sugar apples, fresh	1 medium	0.5	0	0	146	4	15
tangelo, fresh	1 medium	0.1	0	0	39	3	1
tangerine, fresh	1 medium	0.2	0	0	37	3	1
watermelon, fresh	1 cup	0.2	0	0	50	1	3
FRUIT JUICES AND NECTARS							
apple juice	1 cup	0.3	0	0	116	1	7
apricot nectar	1 cup	0.2	0	0	141	1	9
carrot juice	1 cup	0.2	0	0	96	1	65
cranberry juice cocktail							
low cal	1 cup	0	0	0	45	0	3
regular	1 cup	0.1	0	0	147	0	4
cranberry-apple juice	1 cup	0.2	0.2	0	129	1	5
grape juice	1 cup	0.2	0.1	0	155	1	7
grapefruit juice	1 cup	0.3	0	0	96	0	2
lemon juice	2 T	0	0	0	8	0	0
lime juice	2 T	0	0	0	8	0	0
orange juice	1 cup	0.5	0.1	0	111	1	2

Item	Serving	Total Fat (g)	Saturated Fat (g)	Cholesterol (mg)	Calories	Fiber (g)	Sodium (mg)
orange-grapefruit juice	1 cup	0.2	0	0	107	1	8
peach juice or nectar	1 cup	0.1	0	0	134	1	17
pear juice or nectar	1 cup	0	0	0	149	1	9
pineapple juice	1 cup	0.2	0	0	139	1	2
pineapple-orange juice	1 cup	0.1	0	0	125	1	26
prune juice	1 cup	0.1	0	0	181	1	11
tomato juice	1 cup	0.2	0	0	41	2	675
V8 juice	1 cup	0.1	0	0	53	2	600

GRAVIES, SAUCES, AND DIPS

Item	Serving	Total Fat (g)	Saturated Fat (g)	Cholesterol (mg)	Calories	Fiber (g)	Sodium (mg)
au jus, mix	1/2 cup	0.3	0.2	0	24	0	289
barbecue sauce	1 T	0.3	0	0	12	0	127
béarnaise sauce, mix	1/4 pkg.	25.6	15.7	71	263	0	474
beef gravy, canned	1/2 can	3.4	1.7	4	77	0	73
brown gravy							
from mix	1/2 cup	0.1	0	0	4	0	66
hmde	1/4 cup	14.0	NA	NA	164	0	NA
catsup, tomato	1 T	0.1	0	0	16	0	156
chicken gravy							
canned	1/2 can	8.5	2.1	3	118	0	859
from mix	1/2 cup	0.9	0.2	1	41	0	566
giblet from can	1/4 cup	2.0	NA	NA	35	0	320
chili sauce	1 T	0	0	0	16	0	191
dip made with sour							
cream	2 T	4.8	2.5	8	53	0	300
enchilada dip, Frito's	1 oz.	1.2	NA	1	35	0	NA
guacamole dip	1 oz.	12.0	NA	14	108	0	370
hollandaise sauce	1/4 cup	18.5	5.6	160	180	0	332
home-style gravy,							
from mix	1/4 cup	0.5	0.1	1	25	0	374
jalapeño dip	1 oz.	1.1	0.4	60	33	0	120

Item	Serving	Total Fat (g)	Saturated Fat (g)	Cholesterol (mg)	Calories	Fiber (g)	Sodium (mg)
mushroom gravy							
canned	1/2 can	4.0	0.6	0	75	0	849
from mix	1/2 cup	0.4	0.2	0	35	0	701
mushroom sauce, from mix	1/4 pkg.	3.2	1.7	11	71	0	479
mustard							
brown	1 T	0.9	0	0	14	0	200
yellow	1 T	0.7	0	0	11	0	194
onion dip	2 T	4.0	NA	0	60	0	260
onion gravy, from mix	1/2 cup	0.3	0.2	0	40	0	518
pesto sauce, commercial	1 oz.	14.6	NA	NA	155	0	244
picante sauce	6 T	0.6	0	0	48	1	480
pork gravy, from mix	1/2 cup	0.9	0.4	1	38	0	617
sour-cream sauce	1/4 cup	11.9	NA	28	124	0	126
soy sauce	1 T	0	0	0	11	0	1029
soy sauce, reduced sodium	1 T	0	0	0	11	0	600
spaghetti sauce							
"healthy"/"lite" varieties	1/2 cup	1.0	0	0	50	1	350
hmde, w/reg. ground							
beef	1/2 cup	18.7	6.9	32	243	1	505
meat flavor, jar	1/2 cup	6.0	1.0	5	100	1	600
meatless, jar	1/2 cup	1.0	NA	0	70	NA	600
mushroom, jar	1/2 cup	2.0	NA	0	70	NA	500
spinach dip (sour cream							
& mayo)	2 T	7.1	1.8	10	74	1	138
steak sauce							
A-1	1 T	0	0	0	12	0	400
others	1 T	0	0	0	18	0	405
stroganoff sauce, mix	1/4 pkg.	2.9	1.8	10	73	0	493
sweet & sour sauce	1/4 cup	0.2	0	0	131	0	40
tabasco sauce	1 t	0	0	0	1	0	NA
taco sauce	1 T	0	0	0	1	0	52
tartar sauce	1 T	7.9	0	0	70	0	75

Item	Serving	Total Fat (g)	Saturated Fat (g)	Cholesterol (mg)	Calories	Fiber (g)	Sodium (mg)
teriyaki sauce	1 T	0	0	0	15	0	690
turkey gravy							
canned	1/2 can	3.1	0.9	3	76	0	868
from mix	1/2 cup	0.9	0.3	1	43	0	749
white sauce							
thin	2 T	2.6	0.9	4	37	0	100
medium	2 T	4.1	1.8	5	54	1	106
thick	2 T	5.2	2.3	7	65	0	111
Worcestershire sauce	1 T	0	0	0	12	0	244

MEATS (all cooked w/o added fat unless otherwise noted)

beef, extra lean, ≤ 5% fat

Item	Serving	Total Fat (g)	Saturated Fat (g)	Cholesterol (mg)	Calories	Fiber (g)	Sodium (mg)
(cooked)							
Healthy Choice lean							
ground beef	3 1/2 oz.	3.5	0.9	48	114	0	210
round, eye of,							
lean	3 1/2 oz.	4.2	1.5	52	130	0	60
beef, lean, 5-10% fat							
(cooked)							
arm/blade, lean pot							
roast	3 1/2 oz.	9.4	3.5	95	207	0	60
flank steak, fat trimmed	3 1/2 oz.	8.0	2.9	82	193	0	63
hindshank, lean	3 1/2 oz.	9.4	4.0	76	207	0	70
porterhouse steak,							
lean	3 1/2 oz.	10.4	5.3	90	225	0	60
rib steak, lean	3 1/2 oz.	9.4	5.0	80	207	0	70
round							
bottom, lean	3 1/2 oz.	9.4	3.4	96	207	0	51
roasted	3 1/2 oz.	7.4	2.7	81	189	0	64
rump, lean,							
pot-roasted	3 1/2 oz.	7.0	2.5	60	179	0	61
top, lean	3 1/2 oz.	6.4	2.2	89	211	0	60

Item	Serving	Total Fat (g)	Saturated Fat (g)	Cholesterol (mg)	Calories	Fiber (g)	Sodium (mg)
beef, lean, 5-10% fat *(cont.)*							
short plate, sep. lean							
only	3 1/2 oz.	10.4	5.3	90	225	0	60
sirloin steak, lean	3 1/2 oz.	8.9	3.6	76	201	0	67
sirloin tip, lean roasted	3 1/2 oz.	9.4	3.9	90	207	0	62
tenderloin, lean, broiled	3 1/2 oz.	11.1	4.2	83	219	0	60
top sirloin, lean, broiled	3 1/2 oz.	7.9	3.1	89	201	0	60
beef, regular, 11-17.4%							
fat (cooked)							
chuck, separable lean	3 1/2 oz.	15.2	6.2	105	268	0	70
club steak, lean	3 1/2 oz.	12.9	6.1	90	240	0	60
cubed steak	3 1/2 oz.	15.4	3.3	85	264	0	45
hamburger							
extra lean	3 oz.	13.9	6.3	82	253	0	49
lean	3 oz.	15.7	7.2	78	268	0	56
rib roast, lean	3 1/2 oz.	15.2	5.5	85	264	0	75
sirloin tips, roasted	3 1/2 oz.	15.2	3.2	85	264	0	50
stew meat, round, raw	4 oz.	15.3	3.2	85	294	0	50
T-bone, lean only	3 1/2 oz.	10.3	4.2	80	212	0	66
tenderloin, marbled	3 1/2 oz.	15.2	7.0	86	264	0	61
beef, high fat, ≥ 17.5%							
fat (cooked)							
arm/blade, pot-roasted	3 1/2 oz.	26.5	9.3	84	354	0	50
chuck, ground	3 1/2 oz.	23.9	9.6	100	327	0	65
hamburger, regular	3 oz.	19.6	8.2	87	286	0	60
meatballs	1 oz.	5.5	2.0	30	78	0	94
porterhouse steak							
lean & marbled	3 1/2 oz.	19.6	8.2	80	286	0	60
rib steak	3 1/2 oz.	14.7	6.0	81	286	0	62
rump, pot-roasted	3 1/2 oz.	19.6	8.2	80	286	0	60
short ribs, lean	3 1/2 oz.	19.6	8.2	80	286	0	60
sirloin, broiled	3 1/2 oz.	18.7	7.7	78	278	0	63

Item	Serving	Total Fat (g)	Saturated Fat (g)	Cholesterol (mg)	Calories	Fiber (g)	Sodium (mg)
beef, high fat *(cont.)*							
sirloin, ground	3 1/2 oz.	26.5	9.3	84	354	0	50
T-bone, broiled	3 1/2 oz.	26.5	10.5	90	354	0	65
beef, highest fat,							
≥ 27.5% fat (cooked)							
brisket, lean & marbled	3 1/2 oz.	30.0	12.0	85	367	0	55
chuck, stew meat	3 1/2 oz.	30.0	12.0	85	367	0	55
corned, medium fat	3 1/2 oz.	30.2	14.9	75	372	0	1726
rib roast	3 1/2 oz.	30.0	12.0	85	367	0	55
ribeye steak, marbled	3 1/2 oz.	38.8	18.2	90	440	0	60
short ribs	3 1/2 oz.	31.7	10.5	90	382	0	55
steak, chicken fried	3 1/2 oz.	30.0	7.0	120	389	0	370
lamb							
blade chop							
lean	1 chop	6.4	2.7	50	128	0	46
lean & marbled	3 1/2 oz.	26.1	14.8	95	380	0	65
leg							
lean	3 1/2 oz.	8.1	3.4	100	180	0	60
lean & marbled	3 1/2 oz.	14.5	9.0	97	242	0	52
loin chop							
lean	3 1/2 oz.	8.1	4.2	80	180	0	68
lean & marbled	3 1/2 oz.	22.5	11.7	58	302	0	38
rib chop							
lean	3 1/2 oz.	8.1	5.0	50	180	0	60
lean & marbled	3 1/2 oz.	21.2	13.0	70	292	0	30
shoulder							
lean	3 1/2 oz.	9.9	5.3	100	248	0	70
lean & marbled	3 1/2 oz.	27.0	14.9	97	430	0	70
miscellaneous meats							
bacon substitute							
(breakfast strip)	2 strips	4.0	0.8	0	50	0	234
beefalo	3 1/2 oz.	6.3	2.7	58	188	0	82

Item	Serving	Total Fat (g)	Saturated Fat (g)	Cholesterol (mg)	Calories	Fiber (g)	Sodium (mg)
miscellaneous meats *(cont.)*							
frog legs							
cooked	4 large	0.3	NA	57	73	0	NA
flour-coated & fried	6 large	28.6	NA	NA	418	0	NA
rabbit, stewed	3 1/2 oz.	10.1	2.0	60	216	0	35
venison, roasted	3 1/2 oz.	2.5	1.2	111	157	0	54
organ meats							
brains, all kinds, raw	3 oz.	7.4	NA	1701	106	0	106
heart							
beef, lean, braised	3 1/2 oz.	5.7	2.0	195	188	0	65
calf, braised	3 1/2 oz.	9.1	NA	NA	208	0	112
hog, braised	3 1/2 oz.	6.9	1.7	285	195	0	46
kidney, beef, braised	3 1/2 oz.	3.4	1.1	387	144	0	134
liver							
beef, braised	3 1/2 oz.	3.8	1.9	400	140	0	70
beef, pan fried	3 1/2 oz.	10.6	2.8	482	229	0	106
calf, braised	3 1/2 oz.	4.7	2.1	450	140	0	45
calf, pan fried	3 1/2 oz.	13.2	3.4	530	261	0	82
tongue							
beef, etc., pickled	1 oz.	5.7	NA	NA	75	0	NA
beef, etc, potted	1 oz.	6.4	1.5	32	81	0	20
beef, med. fat,							
braised	3 1/2 oz.	16.7	NA	NA	244	0	60
pork							
bacon							
cured, broiled	1 slice	3.1	1.1	5	35	0	101
cured, raw	1 slice	16.2	4.8	15	156	0	152
bacon bits blade							
lean	3 1/2 oz.	9.6	6.1	116	219	0	70
lean, marbled	3 1/2 oz.	18.0	8.4	67	290	0	70
Boston butt							
lean	3 1/2 oz.	14.2	5.3	89	304	0	65

Item	Serving	Total Fat (g)	Saturated Fat (g)	Cholesterol (mg)	Calories	Fiber (g)	Sodium (mg)
pork *(cont.)*							
lean & marbled	3 1/2 oz.	28.0	9.6	88	348	0	65
Canadian bacon,							
broiled	1 oz.	1.8	0.6	14	43	0	360
ham							
cured, butt, lean	3 1/2 oz.	4.5	1.5	38	159	0	1255
cured, butt, lean &							
marbled	3 1/2 oz.	13.0	4.0	60	246	0	900
cured, canned	3 oz.	5.0	1.5	38	120	0	1255
cured, shank, lean	3 1/2 oz.	6.3	3.0	59	176	0	1100
cured, shank, lean &							
marbled	2 slices	13.8	5.0	60	255	0	900
fresh, lean	3 1/2 oz.	6.4	1.5	40	222	0	65
fresh, lean, marbled & fat	3 1/2 oz.	18.3	6.5	85	306	0	65
ham loaf, glazed	3 1/2 oz.	14.7	6.0	116	247	0	811
smoked	3 1/2 oz.	11.0	4.3	51	175	0	800
smoked, 95% lean	3 1/2 oz.	5.5	1.8	53	144	0	800
loin chop							
lean	1 chop	7.7	3.0	55	170	0	40
lean & fat	1 chop	22.5	8.8	90	314	0	63
picnic							
cured, lean	3 1/2 oz.	9.9	4.4	88	211	0	920
fresh, lean	3 1/2 oz.	7.4	3.2	75	150	0	65
shoulder, lean	2 slices	5.4	3.0	70	162	0	50
shoulder, marbled	2 slices	14.3	6.0	60	234	0	30
pig's feet, pickled	1 oz.	4.1	1.3	30	56	0	261
rib chop, trimmed	3 1/2 oz.	9.9	3.5	81	209	0	67
rib roast, trimmed	3 1/2 oz.	10.0	3.6	83	204	0	65
sausage							
brown and serve	1 oz.	9.4	3.1	24	105	0	366
patty	1	8.4	2.9	22	100	0	349
regular link	1/2 oz.	4.7	1.6	15	52	0	170

Item	Serving	Total Fat (g)	Saturated Fat (g)	Cholesterol (mg)	Calories	Fiber (g)	Sodium (mg)
pork *(cont.)*							
sirloin, lean, roasted	3 1/2 oz.	10.2	3.6	85	207	0	70
spareribs roasted	6 medium	35.0	11.8	121	396	0	93
tenderloin, lean, roast	3 1/2 oz.	4.8	1.6	78	155	0	66
top loin chop, trimmed	3 1/2 oz.	7.7	2.7	79	193	0	65
top loin roast, trimmed	3 1/2 oz.	7.5	2.8	77	187	0	65
processed meats							
bacon substitute (breakfast strips)	2 strips	4.0	0.8	0	50	0	234
beef breakfast strips	2 strips	7.2	NA	26	114	0	380
beef, chipped	2 slices	3.6	1.0	24	114	0	1969
beef jerky	1 oz.	4.0	2.4	30	109	0	280
bologna, beef/beef & pork	1 oz.	8.0	3.0	15	85	0	200
bratwurst							
pork	2 oz. link	22.0	7.9	51	256	0	473
pork & beef	2 oz. link	19.5	7.0	44	226	0	778
braunshweiger (pork liver sausage)	1 oz.	7.8	4.9	28	65	0	473
chicken roll	1 oz.	1.3	0.8	10	30	0	112
corn dog	1	20.0	8.4	37	330	0	1252
corned beef, jellied	1 oz.	2.9	1.0	3	31	0	150
ham, chopped	1 oz.	2.3	0.8	17	55	0	625
hot dog/frank							
beef	1	13.2	8.8	27	145	0	504
chicken	1	8.8	2.5	45	116	0	616
97% fat free varieties	1	1.6	0.6	22	55	0	515
turkey	1	8.1	2.7	39	102	0	45
kielbasa (Polish sausage)	1 oz.	8.3	2.0	10	80	0	305
knockwurst/knackwurst	2 oz. link	18.9	3.2	36	209	0	560
liver pâté, goose	1 oz.	12.4	3.3	43	131	0	192

Item	Serving	Total Fat (g)	Saturated Fat (g)	Cholesterol (mg)	Calories	Fiber (g)	Sodium (mg)
processed meats *(cont.)*							
pepperoni	1 oz.	13.0	5.4	NA	148	0	600
pork & beef	1 oz.	9.1	3.3	15	100	0	367
salami							
cooked	1 oz.	10.0	6.6	30	116	0	490
dry/hard	1 oz.	10.0	3.0	16	126	0	400
sausage							
Italian	2 oz. link	17.2	6.1	52	216	0	618
90% fat free varieties	1 oz.	2.3	0.8	19	43	0	250
Polish	1 oz. link	8.1	2.9	20	92	0	248
smoked	2 oz. link	20.0	9.2	48	229	0	642
Vienna	1 sausage	4.0	1.5	8	45	0	152
Spam	1 oz.	7.4	NA	NA	87	0	432
turkey breast	1 oz.	1.5	0.6	12	51	0	21
turkey ham	1 oz.	1.5	0.5	18	36	0	278
turkey loaf	1 oz.	2.7	0.8	14	43	0	278
turkey pastrami	1 oz.	1.8	0.3	15	40	0	270
turkey roll	1 oz.	4.5	1.1	24	72	0	277
turkey salami	1 oz.	3.7	1.1	23	55	0	266
veal							
arm steak							
lean	3 1/2 oz.	4.8	3.0	78	180	0	70
lean & fat	3 1/2 oz.	19.0	9.0	80	298	0	75
blade							
lean	3 1/2 oz.	8.4	3.5	100	228	0	80
lean & fat	3 1/2 oz.	16.6	7.0	100	276	0	80
breast, stewed	3 1/2 oz.	18.6	8.7	100	256	0	70
chuck, med. fat,							
braised	3 1/2 oz.	12.8	6.0	101	235	0	80
cutlet							
breaded	3 1/2 oz.	15.0	NA	NA	319	0	NA
round, lean	3 1/2 oz.	12.8	5.2	102	194	0	90

Item	Serving	Total Fat (g)	Saturated Fat (g)	Cholesterol (mg)	Calories	Fiber (g)	Sodium (mg)
veal *(cont.)*							
round, lean & fat	3 1/2 oz.	15.0	6.8	101	277	0	90
flank, med. fat,							
stewed	3 1/2 oz.	32.0	15.8	101	390	0	80
foreshank, med. fat,							
stewed	3 1/2 oz.	10.4	5.3	101	216	0	80
loin, med. fat,							
broiled	3 1/2 oz.	13.4	5.4	109	234	0	91
loin chop							
lean	1 chop	4.8	3.0	95	149	0	65
lean & fat	3 1/2 oz.	13.3	7.0	101	250	0	80
plate, med. fat,							
stewed	3 1/2 oz.	21.2	10.5	101	303	0	80
rib chop							
lean	1 chop	4.6	3.0	100	125	0	65
lean & fat	1 chop	18.4	6.0	100	264	0	65
rump, marbled,							
roasted	3 1/2 oz.	11.0	6.1	101	225	0	80
sirloin							
lean, roasted	3 1/2 oz.	3.4	1.9	90	175	0	80
marbled, roasted	3 1/2 oz.	6.5	2.9	108	181	0	90
sirloin steak							
lean	3 1/2 oz.	6.0	2.3	108	204	0	90
lean & fat	3 1/2 oz.	20.4	9.1	100	305	0	86

MILK AND YOGURT

Item	Serving	Total Fat (g)	Saturated Fat (g)	Cholesterol (mg)	Calories	Fiber (g)	Sodium (mg)
buttermilk							
1% fat	1 cup	2.2	1.3	9	99	0	257
dry	1 T	0.4	0.2	5	25	0	103
choc. milk							
2% fat	1 cup	5.0	3.1	17	179	0	150
whole	1 cup	8.5	5.3	30	250	0	149

Item	Serving	Total Fat (g)	Saturated Fat (g)	Cholesterol (mg)	Calories	Fiber (g)	Sodium (mg)
condensed milk, sweetened	1/2 cup	14.0	2.1	13	323	0	49
evaporated milk							
skim	1/2 cup	0.4	0	0	97	0	15
whole	1/2 cup	10.0	4.5	27	126	0	99
hot cocoa							
low cal, mix w/water	1 cup	0.8	0.4	2	50	0	231
mix w/water	1 cup	3.0	0.7	5	110	0	149
w/skim milk	1 cup	2.0	0.9	12	158	0	135
w/whole milk	1 cup	9.1	5.6	33	218	0	123
low fat milk							
1/2% fat	1 cup	1.0	0.4	10	90	0	125
1% fat	1 cup	2.6	1.6	10	102	0	123
1.5% fat/acidophilus	1 cup	4.7	2.9	18	122	0	122
2% fat	1 cup	4.7	2.2	18	121	0	122
malt powder	1 T	1.6	0.9	4	86	0	103
malted milk	1 cup	9.9	6.0	37	236	0	223
milkshake							
choc. thick	1 cup	17.2	5.0	32	341	1	333
soft serve	1 cup	7.0	2.3	35	218	1	240
vanilla, thick	1 cup	14.7	5.9	37	274	0	299
Ovaltine, w/1% milk	1 cup	2.8	1.1	33	173	0	201
skim milk							
liquid	1 cup	0.4	0.3	4	86	0	126
nonfat dry powder	1/4 cup	0.2	0.2	6	109	0	161
whole milk							
3.5% fat	1 cup	8.0	4.9	34	150	0	122
dry powder	1/4 cup	8.6	5.4	31	159	0	119
yogurt							
coffee/vanilla, low fat	1 cup	2.8	1.8	11	194	0	149
frzn, low fat	1/2 cup	3.0	2.0	10	115	0	55
frzn, nonfat	1/2 cup	0.2	0	0	81	0	39

Item	Serving	Total Fat (g)	Saturated Fat (g)	Cholesterol (mg)	Calories	Fiber (g)	Sodium (mg)
yogurt *(cont.)*							
fruit flavored, low fat	1 cup	2.6	0.1	10	225	0	121
plain							
low fat	1 cup	3.5	2.3	14	144	0	159
skim (nonfat)	1 cup	0.4	0.3	4	127	0	174
whole milk	1 cup	7.4	4.8	29	139	0	105
MISCELLANEOUS							
Bac o Bits, General Mills	1 T	1.3	NA	0	33	0	130
baking powder	1 t	0	0	0	3	0	426
baking soda	1 t	0	0	0	0	0	821
bouillon cube, beef or							
chicken	1	0.2	0.1	0	8	0	900
chewing gum	1 stick	0	0	0	10	0	0
choc., baking	1 oz.	15.0	8.9	0	143	1	1
cocoa, dry	1/3 cup	3.6	2.2	0	115	2	2
gelatin, dry	1 pkg.	0	0	0	23	0	0
honey	1 T	0	0	0	64	0	1
horseradish, prepared	1 t	0	0	0	2	0	7
icing, decorator	1 t	2.0	0.2	0	70	0	11
jam, all varieties	1 T	0	0	0	54	0	2
jelly, all varieties	1 T	0	0	0	49	0	3
marmalade, citrus	1 T	0	0	0	51	0	3
meat tenderizer	1 t	0	0	0	2	0	1760
molasses	1 T	0	0	0	50	0	3
olives							
black	2 large	4.0	0.6	0	37	1	240
Greek	3 medium	7.1	0.8	0	67	1	631
green	2 medium	1.6	0.2	0	15	0	200
pickle relish							
chow chow	1 oz.	0.4	0	0	8	0	400
sweet	1 T	0.1	0	0	21	0	107

Item	Serving	Total Fat (g)	Saturated Fat (g)	Cholesterol (mg)	Calories	Fiber (g)	Sodium (mg)
pickles							
bread & butter	4 slices	0.1	0	0	18	0	202
dill or sour	1 large	0.2	0	0	11	1	950
Kosher	1 oz.	0.1	0	0	7	0	350
sweet	1 oz.	0.4	0	0	146	0	268
salt	1 t	0	0	0	0	0	2132
Shake & Bake, Gen. Foods	1/4 pkg.	2.6	1.0	0	69	0	600
spices/seasonings	1 t	0.2	0	0	5	0	0
sugar, all varieties	1 T	0	0	0	46	0	0
sugar substitutes	1 packet	0	0	0	4	0	0
syrup, all varieties	1 T	0	0	0	60	0	0
vinegar	1 T	0	0	0	2	0	0
yeast	1 T	0.1	0	0	23	0	10
NUTS AND SEEDS							
almond paste	1 T	4.5	0.4	0	80	1	2
almonds	12 - 15	9.3	1.0	0	104	1	0
Brazil nuts	4 medium	11.5	2.3	0	114	1	0
cashews, roasted	6 - 8	7.8	1.3	0	94	2	2
chestnuts, fresh	3 small	0.8	0	0	66	4	1
coconut, dried,							
shredded	1/3 cup	9.2	10.0	0	135	1	6
hazelnuts (filberts)	10 - 12	10.6	1.0	0	106	1	0
macadamia nuts,							
roasted	6 medium	12.3	2.0	0	117	1	0
mixed nuts							
w/peanuts	8 - 12	10.0	1.5	0	109	2	2
w/o peanuts	2 T	10.1	2.0	0	110	2	2
peanut butter, creamy or							
chunky	1 T	8.0	1.5	0	94	1	75
peanuts							
chopped	2 T	8.9	1.0	0	104	2	3

Item	Serving	Total Fat (g)	Saturated Fat (g)	Cholesterol (mg)	Calories	Fiber (g)	Sodium (mg)
peanuts *(cont.)*							
honey roasted	2 T	8.9	1.5	0	112	2	150
in shell	1 cup	17.7	2.0	0	209	3	156
pecans	2 T	9.1	0.5	0	90	1	0
pine nuts (pignolia)	2 T	9.1	1.5	0	85	2	0
pistachios	2 T	7.7	0.8	0	92	1	1
poppy seeds	1 T	3.8	0.3	0	44	1	3
pumpkin seeds	2 T	7.9	3.0	0	93	1	4
sesame nut mix	2 T	5.1	1.5	0	65	1	165
sesame seeds	2 T	8.8	1.2	0	94	1	6
sunflower seeds	2 T	8.9	1.0	0	102	1	1
trail mix w/seeds, nuts,							
carob	2 T	5.1	0.7	0	87	1	3
walnuts	2 T	7.7	0.3	0	80	1	0
PASTA, NOODLES, AND RICE (all measurements after cooking unless otherwise noted)							
macaroni							
semolina	1 cup	0.7	0	0	159	1	1
whole wheat	1 cup	0.6	0.1	0	183	5	4
noodles							
Alfredo	1 cup	29.7	9.8	73	462	3	844
almondine, from mix	1/4 pkg.	12.0	NA	NA	240	1	700
cellophone, fried	1 cup	4.2	0.6	0	141	0	6
chow mein, canned	1/2 cup	8.0	1.6	0	153	0	210
egg	1 cup	2.4	0.4	50	200	1	3
manicotti	1 cup	0.4	0.1	0	129	1	1
ramen, all varieties	1 cup	6.5	0.9	0	188	1	978
rice	1 cup	0	0	0	140	1	0
romanoff	1 cup	23.0	11.9	95	372	3	774

Item	Serving	Total Fat (g)	Saturated Fat (g)	Cholesterol (mg)	Calories	Fiber (g)	Sodium (mg)
rice							
brown	1/2 cup	0.6	0	0	116	2	0
fried	1/2 cup	7.2	0.7	0	181	1	550
long grain & wild	1/2 cup	2.1	0.2	0	120	2	530
pilaf	1/2 cup	7.0	0.6	0	170	1	600
Spanish style	1/2 cup	2.1	0.1	0	106	1	547
white	1/2 cup	1.2	0	0	111	0	0
spaghetti, enriched	1 cup	1.0	0	0	159	1	1

POULTRY

Item	Serving	Total Fat (g)	Saturated Fat (g)	Cholesterol (mg)	Calories	Fiber (g)	Sodium (mg)
chicken							
breast							
w/skin, fried	1/2 breast	10.7	3.0	87	236	0	77
w/o skin, fried	1/2 breast	6.1	1.5	90	179	0	81
w/skin, roasted	1/2 breast	7.6	2.9	70	193	0	72
w/o skin, roasted	1/2 breast	3.1	1.0	80	142	0	70
fryers							
w/skin, batter							
dipped, fried	3 1/2 oz.	17.4	3.0	95	289	0	85
w/o skin, fried	3 1/2 oz.	11.1	1.0	70	237	0	60
w/skin, roasted	3 1/2 oz.	13.6	3.5	90	239	0	75
w/o skin, roasted	3 1/2 oz.	7.4	1.9	80	190	0	70
giblets, fried	3 1/2 oz.	13.5	3.8	446	277	0	113
gizzard, simmered	3 1/2 oz.	3.7	1.5	393	153	0	58
heart, simmered	3 1/2 oz.	7.9	1.0	194	185	0	67
leg							
w/skin, fried	1 leg	8.7	4.4	99	120	0	92
w/skin, roasted	1 leg	5.8	4.2	105	112	0	99
w/o skin, roasted	1 leg	2.5	0.7	41	76	0	42
liver simmered	3 1/2 oz.	5.5	1.8	631	157	0	51
roll, light meat	3 1/2 oz.	7.4	1.2	60	159	0	662
stewers							

Item	Serving	Total Fat (g)	Saturated Fat (g)	Cholesterol (mg)	Calories	Fiber (g)	Sodium (mg)
w/skin	3 1/2 oz.	18.9	5.1	79	285	0	73
w/o skin	3 1/2 oz.	11.9	3.1	83	237	0	78
thigh							
w/skin, fried	1 thigh	11.3	2.5	60	180	0	55
w/skin, roasted	1 thigh	9.6	2.7	58	153	0	52
w/o skin, roasted	1 thigh	5.7	2.4	75	109	0	95
wing							
w/skin, fried	1 wing	9.1	1.9	26	121	0	25
w/skin, roasted	1 wing	6.6	1.9	29	99	0	28
duck,							
w/skin, roasted	3 1/2 oz.	28.4	9.7	84	337	0	59
w/o skin, roasted	3 1/2 oz.	11.2	4.2	89	201	0	65
pheasant,							
w/ or w/o skin,							
cooked	3 1/2 oz.	9.3	3.0	102	211	0	98
quail, w/o skin,							
cooked	3 1/2 oz.	9.3	3.0	102	213	0	95
turkey							
breast							
barbecued, Louis Rich	3 1/2 oz.	5.0	1.4	56	135	0	860
oven roasted, Louis Rich	3 1/2 oz.	3.0	1.0	35	115	0	786
smoked, Louis Rich	3 1/2 oz.	4.0	0.7	45	120	0	910
dark meat							
w/skin, roasted	3 1/2 oz.	11.5	3.5	89	221	0	76
w/o skin, roasted	3 1/2 oz.	7.2	2.4	85	187	0	79
ground	3 1/2 oz.	14.0	4.0	85	225	0	105
ham, cured	3 1/2 oz.	5.1	1.7	62	128	0	996
light meat							
w/skin, roasted	3 1/2 oz.	8.3	2.3	76	197	0	63
w/o skin, roasted	3 1/2 oz.	3.2	1.0	69	157	0	64

Item	Serving	Total Fat (g)	Saturated Fat (g)	Cholesterol (mg)	Calories	Fiber (g)	Sodium (mg)
turkey *(cont.)*							
loaf, breast meat	3 1/2 oz.	1.6	0.5	41	110	0	431
patties, breaded/fried	1 patty	16.9	2.0	30	266	0	500
roll, light meat	3 1/2 oz.	7.2	2.0	43	147	0	489
sausage, cooked	1 oz.	3.4	1.5	23	50	0	200
sliced w/gravy, frzn	5 oz.	3.7	1.2	26	95	0	706
wing drumettes,							
smoked, Louis Rich	3 1/2 oz.	7.0	1.8	70	165	0	60
SALAD DRESSING							
blue cheese							
fat free	1 T	0	0	0	10	0	140
low cal	1 T	0.8	0	2	11	0	174
regular	1 T	8.0	1.4	0	77	0	156
buttermilk, from mix	1 T	5.8	1.0	5	58	0	138
Caesar	1 T	7.0	0.9	13	70	0	100
French							
creamy	1 T	6.9	1.0	0	70	0	185
fat free	1 T	0	0	0	20	0	120
low cal	1 T	0.9	0.1	1	22	0	128
regular	1 T	6.4	0.8	0	67	0	185
garlic, from mix	1 T	9.2	1.4	0	83	0	173
Green Goddess							
low cal	1 T	2.0	0.4	0	27	0	175
regular	1 T	7.0	1.4	0	68	0	173
honey mustard	1 T	6.6	1.0	0	89	0	32
Italian							
creamy	1 T	4.5	1.4	0	52	0	170
fat free	1 T	0	0	0	6	0	210
low cal	1 T	1.5	0.1	1	16	0	128
regular zesty, from mix	1 T	9.2	1.4	0	85	0	123
Kraft, free	1 T	0	0	0	20	0	120

Item	Serving	Total Fat (g)	Saturated Fat (g)	Cholesterol (mg)	Calories	Fiber (g)	Sodium (mg)
Kraft, reduced cal mayonnaise type	1 T	1.0	0	0	25	0	120
low cal	1 T	1.8	0.3	2	19	0	112
regular	1 T	4.9	0.7	4	57	0	105
oil & vinegar	1 T	7.5	1.5	0	69	0	0
ranch style, prep.							
w/mayo	1 T	5.7	0.7	4	54	0	105
Russian							
low cal	1 T	0.7	0.1	1	23	0	141
regular	1 T	7.8	1.1	0	76	0	133
sesame seed	1 T	6.9	0.9	0	68	0	153
sweet & sour	1 T	0.9	0.3	0	29	0	32
Thousand Island							
fat free	1 T	0	0	0	20	0	135
low cal	1 T	1.6	0.2	2	24	0	153
regular	1 T	5.6	0.9	0	59	0	109

SNACK FOODS

Item	Serving	Total Fat (g)	Saturated Fat (g)	Cholesterol (mg)	Calories	Fiber (g)	Sodium (mg)
bagel chips or crisps	1 oz.	8.8	1.3	0	149	1	140
Bugles	1 oz.	8.0	NA	NA	150	0	150
Cheese Puff balls, Cheetos	1 oz.	10.6	4.8	14	161	0	343
Cheese Puffs, Cheetos	1 oz.	10.0	4.8	14	159	0	348
cheese straws	4 pieces	7.2	6.4	NA	109	0	433
corn chips, Frito's							
light	1 oz.	9.7	0.2	0	144	0	200
regular	1 oz.	9.7	1.0	0	155	0	233
corn nuts, all flavors	1 oz.	4.0	NA	0	120	3.0	200
Cracker Jack	1 oz.	1.0	0	0	114	1	85
Doo-Dads, Nabisco	1/2 cup	6.0	NA	NA	140	1	393
Funyuns	1 oz.	6.4	0.8	0	140	0	250

Item	Serving	Total Fat (g)	Saturated Fat (g)	Cholesterol (mg)	Calories	Fiber (g)	Sodium (mg)
party mix (cereal, pretzels, nuts)	1 cup	23.0	2.0	4	312	3	722
popcorn							
air popped	1 cup	0.3	0	0	23	1	0
caramel	1 cup	4.5	1.3	2	150	1	73
microwave, "lite"	1 cup	1.0	0	0	25	1	35
microwave, plain	1 cup	3.0	0.7	0	47	1	100
microwave, w/butter	1 cup	4.5	1.8	1	61	1	100
popped w/oil	1 cup	2.0	0.5	0	38	1	86
pork rinds, Frito-Lay	1 oz.	9.3	3.7	24	151	0	570
potato chips							
individually	10 chips	8.0	2.6	0	113	0	133
by weight	1 oz.	11.2	2.9	0	159	1	182
barbecue flavor	1 oz.	9.5	2.6	0	149	1	150
light, Pringles	1 oz.	7.8	2.0	0	144	0	152
regular, Pringles	1 oz.	12.9	2.0	0	171	0	215
potato sticks	1 oz.	10.2	2.5	0	152	0	71
pretzels	1 oz.	1.0	0.5	0	110	0	451
rice cakes	1	0.4	0	0	35	0	20
tortilla chips							
Doritos	1 oz.	6.6	1.1	0	139	0	140
no oil, baked	1 oz.	1.4	<1.0	0	110	0	120
Tostitos	1 oz.	7.8	1.1	0	145	0	140
SOUPS							
asparagus							
cream of, w/milk	1 cup	8.2	2.1	10	161	1	982
cream of, w/water	1 cup	4.1	1.0	5	87	1	981
bean							
w/bacon	1 cup	5.9	6.0	3	173	4	952
w/franks	1 cup	7.0	2.0	12	187	3	1092
w/ham	1 cup	8.5	2.0	3	231	3	1800

Item	Serving	Total Fat (g)	Saturated Fat (g)	Cholesterol (mg)	Calories	Fiber (g)	Sodium (mg)
bean soups *(cont.)*							
w/o meat	1 cup	3.0	1.5	2	142	5	940
beef							
broth	1 cup	0.5	0.2	1	33	0	642
chunky	1 cup	5.1	2.6	14	171	2	867
beef barley	1 cup	1.1	0.5	6	72	1	871
beef noodle	1 cup	3.1	1.2	5	84	1	952
black bean	1 cup	1.5	1.2	0	116	2	1198
broccoli, creamy							
w/water	1 cup	2.7	1.0	5	69	1	981
Campbell's Chunky							
w/meat	1 cup	5.1	2.0	30	170	2	887
w/o meat	1 cup	3.7	0.6	0	122	3	1010
Campbell's Healthy Request							
chicken, cream of, w/water	1 cup	2.0	NA	10	70	0	490
mushroom cream of,							
w/water	1 cup	2.0	NA	<5	60	0	460
tomato, w/water	1 cup	2.0	NA	0	90	0	430
canned vegetable type,							
w/o meat	1 cup	2.0	0.7	0	67	1	500
cheese w/milk	1 cup	14.6	9.1	48	230	0	1020
chicken							
chunky	1 cup	6.6	2.0	30	178	2	887
cream of, w/milk	1 cup	11.5	4.6	27	191	0	1046
cream of, w/water	1 cup	7.4	2.1	10	116	0	986
chicken & dumplings	1 cup	5.5	1.3	34	97	0	861
chicken & stars	1 cup	1.8	0.7	5	55	1	875
chicken & wild rice	1 cup	2.3	0.5	7	76	1	815
chicken/beef noodle or veg.	1 cup	3.1	1.2	5	83	1	952
chicken noodle							
chunky	1 cup	6.0	1.4	18	116	2	900
w/water	1 cup	2.5	0.7	7	75	0	1107

Item	Serving	Total Fat (g)	Saturated Fat (g)	Cholesterol (mg)	Calories	Fiber (g)	Sodium (mg)
chicken vegetable							
chunky	1 cup	4.8	1.4	17	167	2	1068
w/water	1 cup	2.8	0.9	10	74	1	944
chicken w/noodles,							
chunky	1 cup	5.0	1.4	19	180	2	850
chicken w/rice							
chunky	1 cup	3.2	NA	NA	127	2	1072
w/water	1 cup	1.9	0.5	7	60	1	814
clam chowder							
Manhattan chunky	1 cup	3.4	2.1	14	133	1	1000
New England	1 cup	6.6	3.6	7	163	1	960
consommé w/ gelatin	1 cup	0	0	0	29	0	637
crab	1 cup	1.5	0.4	10	76	1	1234
dehydrated							
asparagus, cream of	1 cup	1.7	0.3	0	59	0	801
bean w/bacon	1 cup	3.5	1.0	3	105	2	928
beef broth cube	1 cube	0.3	0.1	1	6	0	1358
beef noodle	1 cup	0.8	0.3	2	41	0	1041
cauliflower	1 cup	1.7	0.3	0	68	0	843
chicken, cream of	1 cup	5.3	3.4	3	107	1	1184
chicken broth cube	1 cube	0.2	0.1	1	9	0	1484
chicken noodle	1 cup	1.2	0.3	3	53	0	1284
chicken rice	1 cup	1.4	0.3	3	60	0	980
clam chowder							
Manhattan	1 cup	1.6	0.3	0	65	1	1336
New England	1 cup	3.7	0.6	1	95	0	745
minestrone	1 cup	1.7	0.8	3	79	0	1026
mushroom	1 cup	4.9	0.8	1	96	0	1019
onion							
dry mix	1 pkg.	2.3	0.5	2	115	1	3045
prepared	1 cup	0.6	0.1	0	28	0	848
tomato	1 cup	2.4	0.4	1	102	0	943

Item	Serving	Total Fat (g)	Saturated Fat (g)	Cholesterol (mg)	Calories	Fiber (g)	Sodium (mg)
dehydrated soups *(cont.)*							
vegetable beef	1 cup	1.1	0.6	1	53	0	1000
gazpacho	1 cup	0.5	0.3	0	40	2	1183
hmde or restaurant style							
beer cheese	1 cup	23.1	11.4	50	308	1	725
cauliflower, cream of w/whole milk	1 cup	9.7	3.0	20	165	1	800
celery, cream of, w/whole milk	1 cup	10.6	4.0	32	165	1	1010
chicken broth	1 cup	1.4	0.4	1	38	0	776
clam chowder							
Manhattan	1 cup	2.2	0.4	2	76	2	1808
New England	1 cup	14.0	3.4	5	271	1	914
corn chowder, traditional	1 cup	12.0	4.9	24	251	3	632
fish chowder, w/whole milk	1 cup	13.5	5.3	37	285	1	710
gazpacho, traditional	1 cup	7.0	0.3	0	100	2	1183
hot & sour	1 cup	7.1	1.7	52	134	1	1209
mock turtle	1 cup	15.5	5.3	456	246	2	939
onion, French w/o cheese	1 cup	5.8	0.7	0	93	0	1053
oyster stew, w/whole milk	1 cup	17.7	2.5	14	268	0	980
seafood gumbo	1 cup	3.9	2.7	40	155	3	230
lentil	1 cup	1.0	0.2	0	161	3	1020
minestrone							
chunky	1 cup	2.8	1.5	5	127	2	864
w/water	1 cup	2.5	0.8	3	83	1	1026
mushroom, cream of							

Item	Serving	Total Fat (g)	Saturated Fat (g)	Cholesterol (mg)	Calories	Fiber (g)	Sodium (mg)
condensed	1 can	23.1	10.1	30	313	1	2000
w/milk	1 cup	13.6	5.1	20	203	1	1076
w/water	1 cup	9.0	2.4	2	129	1	1031
mushroom barley	1 cup	2.3	NA	0	76	1	800
mushroom w/beef stock	1 cup	4.0	1.6	7	85	1	970
onion	1 cup	1.7	0.3	0	57	1	1053
oyster stew, w/water	1 cup	3.8	2.5	14	59	1	980
pea							
green, w/water	1 cup	2.9	1.4	0	164	2	987
split	1 cup	0.6	0.2	1	58	1	600
split w/ham	1 cup	4.4	1.8	8	189	1	1008
potato, cream of							
w/milk	1 cup	7.4	1.2	5	157	2	1000
shrimp, cream of, w/milk	1 cup	9.3	3.2	17	165	1	976
tomato							
w/milk	1 cup	6.0	2.9	17	160	1	932
w/water	1 cup	1.9	0.4	0	100	0.5	872
tomato beef w/noodle	1 cup	4.3	1.6	5	140	1	917
tomato bisque w/milk	1 cup	6.6	0.5	4	198	1	1048
tomato rice	1 cup	2.7	0.5	2	120	1	815
turkey, chunky	1 cup	4.4	1.2	9	136	2	923
turkey noodle	1 cup	2.0	0.6	5	69	1	815
turkey vegetable	1 cup	3.0	0.9	2	74	1	905
vegetable, chunky	1 cup	3.7	0.6	0	122	2	1010
vegetable w/beef, chunky	1 cup	3.0	1.3	8	134	2	1340
vegetable w/beef broth	1 cup	1.9	0.4	2	81	1	810
vegetarian vegetable	1 cup	1.9	0.3	0	72	1	823
wonton	1 cup	2.0	NA	NA	92	1	878
VEGETABLES							
alfalfa sprouts, raw	1/2 cup	0.1	0	0	5	0	0
artichoke, boiled	1 medium	0.2	0	0	53	3	42

Item	Serving	Total Fat (g)	Saturated Fat (g)	Cholesterol (mg)	Calories	Fiber (g)	Sodium (mg)
artichoke hearts, boiled	1/2 cup	0.1	0	0	37	3	55
asparagus, cooked	1/2 cup	0.3	0.1	0	22	2	4
avocado							
California	1 (6 oz.)	30.0	4.5	0	306	4	21
Florida	1 (11 oz.)	27.0	5.3	0	339	4	14
bamboo shoots, raw	1/2 cup	0.2	0.1	0	21	2	3
beans							
all types, cooked							
w/o fat	1/2 cup	0.4	0.2	0	124	9	1
baked, brown sugar &							
molasses	1/2 cup	1.5	0.2	0	132	4	516
baked, vegetarian	1/2 cup	0.6	0.3	0	235	5	1008
baked w/pork & tomato							
sauce	1/2 cup	1.3	0.5	8	123	5	556
homestyle, canned	1/2 cup	1.6	0.3	0	132	5	550
beets, pickled	1/2 cup	0.1	0	0	75	4	301
black-eyed peas							
(cowpeas), cooked	1/2 cup	0.5	0.1	0	99	2	3
broccoli							
cooked	1/2 cup	0.4	0	0	46	7	16
frzn, chopped, cooked	1/2 cup	0.3	0.1	0	25	2	18
frzn in butter sauce	1/2 cup	2.3	NA	NA	51	2	296
frzn w/cheese sauce	1/2 cup	6.2	1.7	5	116	1	417
raw	1/2 cup	0.2	0	0	12	1	12
brussels sprouts,							
cooked	1/2 cup	0.3	0	0	30	2	17
butter beans,							
canned	1/2 cup	0.6	0	0	100	4	434
cabbage							
Chinese, raw	1 cup	0.2	0	0	10	2	23
green, cooked	1/2 cup	0.2	0	0	16	2	14
red, raw, shredded	1/2 cup	0.1	0	0	10	2	4

Item	Serving	Total Fat (g)	Saturated Fat (g)	Cholesterol (mg)	Calories	Fiber (g)	Sodium (mg)
carrot							
cooked	1/2 cup	0.1	0	0	35	2	52
raw	1 large	0.2	0	0	32	2	25
cauliflower							
cooked	1 cup	0.2	0	0	30	3	4
frzn w/cheese sauce	1/2 cup	6.1	NA	NA	114	2	446
raw	1 cup	0.2	0	0	12	4	7
celery							
cooked	1/2 cup	0.1	0	0	11	1	48
raw	1 stalk	0.1	0	0	6	1	35
chard, cooked	1/2 cup	0.1	0	0	18	2	158
chilies, green	1/4 cup	0	0	0	14	0	3
Chinese-style vegetables,							
frzn	1/2 cup	4.7	0	0	79	3	120
chives, raw, chopped	1 T	0	0	0	1	0	0
collard greens, cooked	1/2 cup	0.1	0	0	13	2	36
corn							
corn on the cob	1 medium	0.9	0.1	0	83	4	4
cream style, canned	1/2 cup	0.4	0.1	0	93	4	365
frzn, cooked	1/2 cup	0.2	0	0	67	4	4
frzn w/ butter sauce	1/2 cup	2.6	NA	NA	105	4	275
whole kernel,							
cooked	1/2 cup	1.1	0.2	0	89	5	14
cucumber							
w/skin	1/2 medium	0.1	0	0	8	1	1
w/o skin, sliced	1/2 cup	0.1	0	0	7	0	1
dandelion greens,							
cooked	1/2 cup	0.3	0	0	17	2	23
eggplant, cooked	1/2 cup	0.1	0	0	13	2	1
endive lettuce	1 cup	0.1	0	0	8	1	6
garbanzo beans							
(chick peas), cooked	1/2 cup	2.1	0.2	0	134	5	6

Item	Serving	Total Fat (g)	Saturated Fat (g)	Cholesterol (mg)	Calories	Fiber (g)	Sodium (mg)
green beans							
french style, cooked	1/2 cup	0.1	0	0	18	2	1
snap, cooked	1/2 cup	0.1	0	0	22	2	2
hominy, white or yellow,							
cooked	1 cup	0.7	0	0	138	3	708
Italian-style vegetables,							
frzn	1/2 cup	7.0	0	0	130	2	489
kale, cooked	1/2 cup	0.3	0	0	21	2	15
kidney beans, red,							
cooked	1/2 cup	0.5	0	0	112	8	2
leeks, chopped, raw	1/4 cup	0.1	0	0	16	1	5
lentils, cooked	1/2 cup	0.4	0	0	116	8	2
lettuce, leaf	1 cup	0.2	0	0	10	1	6
lima beans, cooked	1/2 cup	0.4	0.1	0	108	5	2
miso							
(soybean product)	1/2 cup	8.0	1.2	0	284	4	5032
mushrooms							
canned	1/2 cup	0.2	0	0	19	1	500
fried/sautéed	4 medium	7.4	NA	NA	78	1	NA
raw	1/2 cup	0.2	0	0	9	1	0
mustard greens,							
cooked	1/2 cup	0.4	0	0	13	2	11
okra, cooked	1/2 cup	0.1	0	0	25	3	4
onions							
canned, french-fried	1 oz.	15.0	6.9	0	175	0	334
chopped, raw	1/2 cup	0.2	0	0	27	1	2
parsley, chopped, raw	1/4 cup	0	0	0	5	0	12
parsnips, cooked	1/2 cup	0.2	0	0	63	3	8
peas, green, cooked	1/2 cup	0.2	0	0	67	4	2
pepper, bell, chopped,							
raw	1/2 cup	0.2	0	0	12	2	2
pimentos, canned	1 oz.	0	0	0	10	0	5

Item	Serving	Total Fat (g)	Saturated Fat (g)	Cholesterol (mg)	Calories	Fiber (g)	Sodium (mg)
potato							
au gratin							
from mix	1/2 cup	6.0	3.1	6	140	2	538
hmde	1/2 cup	9.3	5.8	29	160	1	528
baked w/skin	1 medium	0.2	0.1	0	220	4	16
boiled w/o skin	1/2 cup	0.1	0	0	116	2	7
french fries							
frzn	10 pieces	4.4	2.1	0	111	2	15
hmde	10 pieces	8.3	2.5	0	158	1	108
hash browns	1/2 cup	10.9	3.4	23	163	2	101
knishes	1	3.2	0.8	15	73	1	83
mashed							
from flakes, w/milk &							
marg	1/2 cup	6.0	1.6	4	124	1	365
w/milk & marg.	1/2 cup	4.4	1.1	2	111	1	309
pan fried, O'Brien	1/2 cup	12.1	1.5	7	157	3	421
potato pancakes	1 cake	12.6	3.4	93	495	1	388
potato puffs, frzn,							
prep. w/oil	1/2 cup	11.6	3.2	0	183	3	462
scalloped							
from mix	1 serving	5.9	3.6	10	127	1	467
hmde	1/2 cup	4.8	2.8	14	105	1	409
w/cheese	1/2 cup	9.7	NA	NA	177	1	370
twice-baked potato,							
w/cheese	1 medium	9.9	3.3	10	180	1	55
pumpkin, canned	1/2 cup	0.3	0.2	0	41	4	6
radish, raw	10	0.2	0	0	7	1	9
rhubarb, raw	1 cup	0.2	0	0	29	2	2
sauerkraut, canned	1/2 cup	0.2	0	0	22	4	780
scallions, raw	5 medium	0.2	0	0	45	4	1
soybeans, mature,							
cooked	1/2 cup	7.7	1.1	0	149	4	0

Item	Serving	Total Fat (g)	Saturated Fat (g)	Cholesterol (mg)	Calories	Fiber (g)	Sodium (mg)
spinach							
cooked	1/2 cup	0.2	0.1	0	21	3	29
creamed	1/2 cup	5.7	0.8	1	89	3	312
raw	1 cup	0.2	0	0	12	3	22
squash							
acorn							
baked	1/2 cup	0.1	0	0	57	4	4
mashed w/o fat	1/2 cup	0.2	0	0	41	3	3
butternut, cooked	1/2 cup	0.1	0	0	41	4	4
summer							
cooked	1/2 cup	0.3	0	0	18	2	1
raw, slice	1/2 cup	0.1	0	0	13	1	1
winter, cooked	1/2 cup	0.6	0.1	0	39	4	1
succotash, cooked	1/2 cup	0.8	0.1	0	111	3	16
sweet potato							
baked	1 small	0.1	0	0	118	7	12
candied	1/2 cup	3.8	1.4	8	192	5	73
mashed w/o fat	1/2 cup	0.5	0	0	172	5	107
tempeh (soybean product)	1/2 cup	6.4	0.9	0	165	1	5
tofu (soybean curd), raw,							
firm	4 oz.	5.4	0.8	0	86	1	8
tomato							
boiled	1/2 cup	0.3	0	0	30	1	13
raw	1 medium	0.3	0	0	24	1	10
stewed	1/2 cup	0.2	0	0	34	1	325
tomato paste, canned	1/2 cup	1.2	0.2	0	110	4	86
turnip greens, cooked	1/2 cup	0.2	0	0	15	2	21
turnips, cooked	1/2 cup	0.1	0	0	14	2	21
water chestnuts, canned,							
sliced	1/2 cup	0	0	0	35	1	6
watercress, raw	1/2 cup	0	0	0	2	0	7
wax beans, canned	1/2 cup	0.2	0	0	25	2	321

Item	Serving	Total Fat (g)	Saturated Fat (g)	Cholesterol (mg)	Calories	Fiber (g)	Sodium (mg)
yam, boiled/baked	1/2 cup	0.1	0	0	79	3	6
zucchini, cooked	1/2 cup	0.1	0	0	14	2	1

VEGETABLE SALADS

Item	Serving	Total Fat (g)	Saturated Fat (g)	Cholesterol (mg)	Calories	Fiber (g)	Sodium (mg)
Caesar salad w/o anchovies	1 cup	7.2	1.5	19	80	1	145
carrot-raisin salad	1/2 cup	3.7	1.2	49	157	4	762
chef salad w/o dressing	1 cup	4.3	2.0	39	71	1	281
coleslaw							
w/mayo-type dressing	1/2 cup	14.2	0.2	5	147	1	14
w/vinaigrette	1/2 cup	5.5	0	0	77	1	50
gelatin salad w/fruit & cheese	1/2 cup	4.6	0	0	74	0	82
macaroni salad w/mayo	1/2 cup	12.8	2.5	12	200	1	157
pasta primavera salad	1 cup	5.9	0.8	0	149	3	639
potato salad							
German style	1/2 cup	3.5	NA	NA	140	1	NA
w/mayo dressing	1/2 cup	11.5	1.8	85	189	1	662
salad bar items							
alfalfa sprouts	2 T	0	0	0	2	0	0
bacon bits	1 T	1.6	0	6	27	0	181
beets, pickled	2 T	0	0	0	18	0	74
broccoli, raw	2 T	0	0	0	3	0	3
carrots, raw	2 T	0	0	0	6	0	5
cheese, shredded	2 T	4.6	2.5	15	56	0	87
chickpeas	2 T	0.4	0	0	21	1	75
cottage cheese	1/2 cup	5.1	1.5	17	116	0	458
croutons	1/2 oz.	3.0	0.2	0	60	0	189
cucumber	2 T	0	0	0	2	0	0
eggs, cooked, chopped	2 T	1.9	1.0	93	27	0	23
lettuce	1/2 cup	0	0	0	4	0	1
mushrooms, raw	2 T	0	0	0	2	0	0

Item	Serving	Total Fat (g)	Saturated Fat (g)	Cholesterol (mg)	Calories	Fiber (g)	Sodium (mg)
salad bar items *(cont.)*							
onion, raw	2 T	0.1	0	0	7	0	0
pepper, green, raw	2 T	0	0	0	3	0	0
potato salad	1/2 cup	10.3	1.8	85	179	0	661
tomato, raw	2 slices	0	0	0	2	0	1
seven-layer salad	1 cup	17.8	6.1	105	226	2	336
tabbouli salad	1/2 cup	9.5	1.4	0	173	3	542
taco salad w/taco sauce	1 cup	14.0	6.4	41	202	2	404
three-bean salad	1/2 cup	11.2	1.7	0	145	3	307
three-bean salad, w/o oil	1/2 cup	0.3	0	0	90	3	894
Waldorf salad w/mayo	1/2 cup	12.7	2.8	11	157	2	123

ADDITIONAL ITEMS

	Total Fat (g)	Saturated Fat (g)	Cholesterol (mg)	Calories	Fiber (g)	Sodium (mg)

ADDITIONAL ITEMS

	Total Fat (g)	Saturated Fat (g)	Cholesterol (mg)	Calories	Fiber (g)	Sodium (mg)

ADDITIONAL ITEMS

	Total Fat (g)	Saturated Fat (g)	Cholesterol (mg)	Calories	Fiber (g)	Sodium (mg)

The Low Fat Good Food Cookbook by **Martin Katahn**
The chef's bible for low fat cooking

Available wherever books are sold, or if you prefer to order direct, please use the coupon below.